EARLY DIAGNOSIS
OF SPINAL TUMOURS

with surgical technique notes

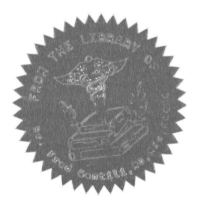

ALDO FORTUNA

LUIGI FERRANTE   PIERPAOLO LUNARDI   MICHELE ACQUI

Early diagnosis of spinal tumours

with surgical technique notes

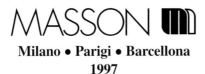

MASSON

Milano • Parigi • Barcellona
1997

Masson S.p.A.   Via F.lli Bressan 2, 20126 Milano
Masson S.A.   120, Bd Saint-Germain, 75280 Paris, Cedex 06
Masson S.A.   Ronda General Mitre 149, 08022 Barcelona

Authors

ALDO
FORTUNA M.D.

Chairman of the 2nd Chair of Neurosurgery
Director of the Neurosurgery Specialization School
Department of Neurological Sciences
University of Rome "La Sapienza"

LUIGI
FERRANTE M.D.

Assistant Professor - 2nd Chair of Neurosurgery
Lecturer of Operative Technique,
Neurosurgery Specialization School
Department of Neurological Sciences
University of Rome "La Sapienza"

PIERPAOLO
LUNARDI M.D.

Assistant Professor - 2nd Chair of Neurosurgery
Lecturer of Stereotactic and Functional Neurosurgery,
Neurosurgery Specialization School
Department of Neurological Sciences
University of Rome "La Sapienza"

MICHELE
ACQUI M.D.

Assistant Neurosurgeon - 2nd Chair of Neurosurgery
Department of Neurological Sciences
University of Rome "La Sapienza"

Preface

In 1925 Elsberg wrote: "... in the 37 years that have passed since Horsley's intervention (1887), our knowledge in the field of the symptomatology of spinal cord tumours and their surgical treatment has made considerable progress...; it is perhaps possible to predict that the day will shortly arrive when the first symptoms and signs of a spinal cord tumour will be so well understood that diagnosis, localization and its removal will be possible at a stage in which only mild paresis and slight sensory disturbances have occurred".

It must be asked if Elsberg's prediction has become a reality today: i.e. if early diagnosis of spinal cord tumours is a usual rather than sporadic occurrence.

The present contribution is the result of such a consideration.

Back in 1964, in a study presented at the XVI Congress of Italian Neurosurgical Society on "Intramedullary Tumours", we first outlined an early syndrome in intramedullary gliomas (A. Fortuna: Diagnostica clinica, *pp. 155-264;* Sindrome precoce, *pp. 202-208 in: Guidetti et al. 1964).*

We hope and believe that the project will prove useful, particularly in view of the fact that new neuroradiological procedures (CT and MRI) are now able to resolve diagnostic uncertainties, making it essential to recognize and interpret the first signs of the early syndrome.

THE AUTHORS

Contents

Introduction

It is common knowledge that there exists a stage of the disease in which clinical features are scarce, with a number of insidious aspects, but in which an instrumental diagnosis, almost always the most useful, can be easily given on condition that a diagnostic suspicion arises. This is particularly important for the neurosurgical clinic, in which an early diagnostic suspicion means, in most cases, a timely diagnosis. The result is a drastic reduction in morbidity and thus a marked improvement in the quality of life.

The following pages describe the initial clinical syndrome, and space will be given both to the patient's voice and the doctor's efforts to recognize and evaluate a particular symptom suggesting a particular diagnostic exam.

Reflecting on a symptom, a sign, or an initial clinical syndrome, and interpreting it correctly is, in our opinion, the only way in which a spinal tumour can reach the neurosurgeon at an initial and non-advanced stage.

Frequency, gender, age, length of the disease

Frequency. More than 70% of neoplastic spinal cord compressions consists of meningiomas, neurinomas and intramedullary tumours; 30% is extradural malignancy. In childhood and adolescence incidences are different since meningiomas (4%), neurinomas (8%), metastasis (4.9%), and lipomas (4.12%) are rare; less rare are the dysembryogenetic tumours (dermoid and epidermoid: 11.2%; theratomas: 2.75%); more frequent are gliomas (24-25%); intramedullary and extradural tumours are more common and 45-50% of them is malign.

Gender. There is a clear predominance of meningiomas in females (75-85%). The greater frequency in males of gliomas (60%), extradural malignancy (62%) and of neurinomas (55%) is clinically insignificant.

Age. The average age is more advanced in meningiomas and extradural malignancy (51 years) than for neurinomas (40 years) and intramedullary tumours (35 years), but if we consider age by decades in relation to gender, these values change and are thus of small diagnostic utility: i.e., in females meningiomas are the most frequent tumours beyond the age of 50.

Duration of the disease. The duration of the disease is of no assistance in assuring an early diagnosis. Indeed, excluding long-term intramedullary tumours, the duration of the simptomatology changes relatively little among gliomas, meningiomas, neurinomas, and the rare benign extradural tumours.

General syndrome

Neoplastic spinal lesions are one of the most important chapters in neurosurgery: the removal of generally benign tumours affecting the spinal cord has been one of the most advanced and impressive stages in neurological surgery since 1887 when the English surgeon Horsley first removed a spinal tumour following the indications of Gowers, a neurologist expert in spinal pathology.

Under the term "spinal cord compression" are grouped all the pathological processes which involve the spinal cord, its covers and roots: the various pathological processes which vary from vertebral malformation to neoplastic disease and to the flogistic thickness of dura, to parasite lesions, all of which involve a similarly mechanical action on the close nervous formations.

The more frequent causes of spinal cord compression are spinal tumours, the degenerative osteo-ligamentous diseases of the vertebral column, and spinal traumas.

What characterizes spinal compression, and in particular that caused by spinal tumours, is its evolution, which is progressive both in time and space: disturbances manifest themselves one after the other, gradually constituting a clinical syndrome revealing that all nervous structures are affected; another feature is that each disturbance increases in intensity. Spinal cord damage thus occurs through a progressive mechanical action, which is either direct in the point of compression or indirect by vascular ischemic phenomena or venous engorgement.

What should be underlined is the remarkable resistance of the nervous structures to this slow compression: lesions are reversible for a long time, as is proved by a paradoxal aspect: a tumour can erode and enlarge the bone walls of spinal canal before irreversible medullary lesions occur.

The general syndrome of spinal cord compression is schematically based on pain, weakness, hypoesthesia and sphincter disturbances, symptoms which can be divided into two groups:

   a) lesional;
   b) sublesional, indicating that long tracts are involved.

Lesional symptoms can be represented by:

- radicular sensory syndrome;
- radicular motor syndrome;
- metameric medullary syndrome, the result of damage to the grey substance (anterior and posterior horns) whose symptoms and signs are difficult to differentiate from radicular ones.

Sublesional symptoms, the consequence of damage to the white substance, cause the long-tract medullary syndrome that consists principally of pyramidal, spinothalamic and posterior funiculi lesions.

Symptoms and signs

In most spinal tumours the first symptom consists of vertebral, radicular or cordonal pain, followed, in order of frequency, by weakness, sensory disturbances (paresthesia, hypoesthesia), sphincteric and neurovegetative disorders, neurogenic claudicatio intermittens, and subarachnoid haemorrhage.

Pain

Vertebral pain or rachiodynia: this can be the only symptom to initiate the clinical pattern and is often associated with radicular or cordonal pain. It is perceived as an aching, deep, and indeterminate pain, limited to two or three contiguous vertebral segments, variable in intensity and perceived in the occipito-cervical, subscapular, dorsal or lumbar regions. Often subcontinuous, it is exacerbated by vertebral flexion, extension or rotation and by those conditions that increase endorachidial pressure (coughing, sneezing, Valsalva's monoeuvre); it is usually associated with an antalgic contracture of the paravertebral muscles. The vertebral pain caused by percussion of the spinous process is more pronounced in extradural malignancy. This first symptom is short, quickly followed (3-6 months) in most cases by cordonal or radicular weakness or by paresthesias or hypoesthesias.

The pathogenesis of vertebral pain is linked with tumoral compression on the osseous and articular structures of the spinal column. While the internal portion of the intervertebral disc lacks nociceptors (McCullock 1989), such structures have been studied in the posterior longitudinal ligament, in the external portion of the anulus, in the articular capsule of the facet-joints and in the anterior aspect of the dura (Yoshizawa et al. 1980). It is probable that the distension of the dura mater can cause vertebral pain in intramedullary tumours, while in extradural ones it is caused by stimulation of osteo-ligamentous nociceptors.
The nociceptive sensations pass in Luschka's sinus-vertebral nerve, a recurrent branch of

the anterior primary trunk which innervates the anterior spinal dural and osteo-ligamentous structure.

Radicular pain: this is localized in the dermatomic area of a sensitive root, and it is a subcontinuous, gnawing ache, with sudden, sharp spasms; it becomes more serious with intrarachidial hypertension and root traction. This pain is characteristic of intradural, extramedullary tumours, forming the initial symptom in 60-70% of cases (Cassinari and Bernasconi 1961; Malik et al. 1991), while it is rarer in extradural (when the tumour involves one or more interpeduncular foramina) and intramedullary tumours (10-15%), when it is more frequent in the lumbosacral gliomas (Broager 1953; Guidetti and Fortuna 1964). Radicular pain can also have a medullary origin, i.e. cornual, in relation to posterior horns excitation.

The pathogenesis of radicular pain is intuitive for extradural and intradural-extramedullary tumours, whereas in intramedullary tumours radicular pain is due, as we have seen, to the grey substance of posterior horn excitation (Antoni 1920; Foerster 1936; Elsberg 1941; Richardson 1960; Guidetti and Fortuna 1964): cornual pain is perceived as burning, stinging, biting, and tearing, with a distribution which is not strictly radicular. It can also appear as sciatica (with negativity of the straight-leg-raising test as in our and other series) or inguinal neuralgia. In our experience no cervical glioma has begun with a radicular pain. The hypothesis that the radicular pain in intramedullary tumours is due to radicular compression by enlarged cord (Shenkin and Alpers 1944) may be sustainable in surgical cases, but it is certainly not so in the initial stage of the disease. It is almost always a monoradicular, not pluriradicular pain, as would be expected from direct compressive action caused by an intramedullary tumour involving a root-bordered, medullary tract.

Cordonal pain: in spinal tumours the cordonal pain is reported as a painful disturbance, or a diffuse burning and sometimes as a sudden and sharp spasm which can last some minutes and leave deep, residual pain in the affected site. It is never of radicular distribution (Elsberg 1941) but spreads indistinctly in a segment of a limb, in a whole limb, or in more limbs; in a part of, half of, or in the whole body.
Cordonal pain is rare in extradural malignancy (3.2%: Torma 1957), although more frequent in intramedullary gliomas, especially when bilateral, than in neurinomas and meningiomas, both at the beginning and, above all, during the evolution of the disease. In intramedullary gliomas, cordonal pain is more frequent in dorsal and cervical cases (Shenkin and Alpers 1944; Guidetti, Fortuna et al. 1964: 50%); an important aspect is its slow and progressively descending distribution, never observed in the extramedullary tumours of our series.

The origin of this pain is almost certainly medullary (Foerster 1932; Austin 1960; Guidetti, Fortuna et al. 1964). Foerster observed that stimulation of the spinothalamic tract provoked pain in the contralateral part of the body under the stimulated myelomere, while the posterior tract stimulation triggered a sharp homolateral pain. By stimulating the posterior cordonal tracts of patients operated on in local anesthesia, Guidetti and Austin (1958 and 1960 respectively) caused a pain like an electric shock, homolateral to the stimulated tract. This particular pain is observed both in extra- and intradural compression (Guidetti 1958; Ectors 1960) and in intramedullary same, where it is more frequent (Guidetti, Fortuna et al. 1964).

Motor deficiency

This is the first and most frequent symptom after the pain, and is described as weakness, exhaustion, and numbness of one or more limbs, at their distal or proximal extremities. Fasciculations are rarely present. Motor disturbances can be due to the damage of one or more anterior roots, to the direct or indirect involvement of the anterior horns (ischemic damage), or to intrinsic or extrinsic compression of the corticospinal tracts. Flaccid motor deficiency results in the first two cases, and spastic in the third, although both can coexist.

The weakness usually starts from the compression site, in relation to the somatotopic disposition of motor fibres of the cruciate pyramidal tract (after crossing the fibres for the lower limbs they are more external, and those for the upper limbs more internal); the development of motor deficiency is thus ascending in extramedullary tumours and descending in intramedullary same, affecting the more cranial muscles (Elsberg 1941; Cassinari and Bernasconi 1961).

Motor deficiency is rare at the start of extradural malignancy (4%) and in 2/3 of cases develops into flaccid paralysis (Torma 1957). In Torma's 214 cases with motor deficiency, 17% had flaccid paralysis in one or two days. In 18% of Arseni et al.'s cases (1959) of vertebral tumour (the series also included benign cases) an acute transverse lesion was present, aspects which are to be considered characteristic of this tumour (Paillas 1963). It should also be noted that forms of apoplexy or sudden deterioration, although unusual, are also noted in intramedullary tumours (Guidetti, Fortuna et al. 1964; Frugoni et al. 1967) and are caused by sudden edema or intra-tumoral haemorrhage or malignant degeneration of the tumour (Guidetti and Carloni 1955), as in glioblastomas (Sloof et al. 1964; Chigasachy and Pennybacker 1968; Fortuna and Giuffrè 1961). Extremely rapid evolution is also described in some cases of extradural meningiomas (Fortuna et al. 1969), and is not so rare as might be thought (Elsberg 1941: 4.3%; Arseni and Ionesco 1958: 7%; 5% in our series). Evolution of this kind is exceptional in neurinomas. A case of thoracic neurinoma with acute transverse lesion by intra-tumoral haemorrhage was reported by Fortuna and La Torre in 1967.

In Nittner's 404 tumours (1976), including cono-caudal tumours (13%), the diagnosis was made at the start of weakness as a first symptom in only 6% of cases. As a rule the weakness in neurinomas, meningiomas, gliomas and in some extradural malignant or benign tumours has a slow and progressive evolution, sometimes with temporary remissions; this feature is more frequent in vertebral angiomas with medullary compression (Fortuna and Guidetti 1961).

The great sensitivity of the pyramidal tract to a direct mechanical action, the great vulnerability of motor cells of the anterior horns to ischemia, and the compression of a motor root, can explain the high rate (70%) of motor deficiency as a first or second symptom at a relatively early stage.

Paresthesias

Like pain, motor deficiencies and hypoesthesias, paresthesias can have radicular (or cornual) and cordonal, mono- or bilateral distribution (Dusser and Barenne 1913; Foerster 1936).

Paresthesias are persistent sensations perceived, without a triggering event, as sensations of tingling, pricking, numbness, or heat and cold. They spread over the thorax, abdomen, and along one or more limbs.

As isolated initial symptoms, they are unusual: 7% in extradural malignancy (Torma 1957), 9% in neurinomas (Broager 1953; Torma 1957), 6.5% in intramedullary gliomas (Guidetti, Fortuna et al. 1964). In meningiomas they constitute, after pain, the most frequent type of initial symptom (27%: Oddsson 1947; 23%: Torma 1957; 37%: Davis and Washburn 1970) and are mainly cordonal, of distal origin. Elsberg (1941) considered paresthesias to have ascending progression in extramedullary tumours, and descending in intramedullary same. In gliomas the progression can be irregular: centripetal at first, from the extremity to the root of a limb (from our series: in a cervical ependymoma there were paresthesias from the dorsal part of the fingers, bilateral and cordonal, to the upper limbs; monolateral and with uncertain distribution in two cases of cervico-dorsal ependymomas, from the first three fingers; and lumbosacral-caudal astrocytomas from the toes) and after centrifugal at the contralateral limb. It has not been noticed in extramedullary tumours (Guidetti, Fortuna et al. 1964).

Sensory deficiency

A spinal tumour rarely starts with a symptom of this kind (3.3% in tumours and vascular malformation, always monolateral; 8% in benign extramedullary tumours and in no cases of extradural malignancy: on average 5.4%, Cassinari and Bernasconi 1961).

Sensory deficiencies are reported by the patient as a reduction of sensory discrimination, "dead skin" sensitivity, or the loss of feeling in a finger, in a limb or in a part of it. They can consist of hypoesthesia or anesthesia, and involve deep and/or surface sensitivity, sometimes with tabetic and syringomyelic modalities.

They can be metameric, due to cornual or radicular involvement (2% of cases in the precocious stage), present a superior level, or be suspended in the case of cordonal compromise (3.6% of cases in the initial stage).

The disposition of fibres in the spino-thalamic tract explains the first extension to the distal dermatomes and the ascending evolution of the sensory deficiency in extramedullary tumours, and descending in intramedullary ones, with, in the latter case, damage to the dermatomes closest to the tumour (Tilney and Elsberg 1926; Kernohan et al. 1931; Shenkin and Alpers 1944; Broager 1953; Guidetti and Carloni 1955; Austin 1960). In 1941 Elsberg had already noticed that an anterior median extramedullary tumour can provoke important sensory disturbance in nearer dermatomes, while leaving intact the sacral ones. In foramen magnum tumours (meningiomas and neurinomas), the superficial sensations and the position sense are more frequently compromised in the upper limbs than in the lower, particularly when homolateral to the tumour (Dodge et al. 1956; Stein et al. 1963). In an intramedullary glioma we can have an ascending progression of the sensory deficiency (Guidetti, Fortuna et al. 1964).

It should be underlined that metameric hypo-anesthesia is more frequent in precocious phases and, for a better diagnosis, must be searched for anamnestically because further progression may conceal it; it constitutes the most important sign of intramedullary lesion, if not pathognomonic (Guidetti, Fortuna et al. 1964); metameric hypo-anesthesia has seldom been noted in extramedullary compression, although less rarely in spondylogenetic myelopathy (Guidetti and Fortuna 1967). Cordonal anesthesia was the first symptom in 6% of intradural extramedullary benign tumours and has never been found, as the first symptom, in intramedullary and extradural tumours.

Sphincteric disturbances

These are rare as the initial symptom both in extramedullary and intramedullary benign tumours (Shenkin and Alpers 1944: in one case of intramedullary astrocytoma they were associated with motor weakness; Broager 1955: in a dorsal glioma they were associated with vertebral pain; in a lumbar glioma they were associated with a vertebral pain and with a radicular pain in a lower limb; Torma 1957; Cassinari and Bernasconi 1961: 1%; Sloof et al. 1964: a high dorsal glioma with bowel and bladder disturbances, a dorsal ependymoma and a cervico-dorsal; Guidetti, Fortuna et al. 1964: a lumbosacral astrocytoma with bladder disturbance treated for a long time in a variety of ways; Gautier-Smith 1967). In conus medullaris tumours they are usual at the start of clinical history (Norstrom et al. 1961; Rewcastre and Berry 1964; Cassinari and Bernasconi 1961: in 16.6% of vascular tumours and malformations and in 8-9% of extradural malignancy).

Sexual disturbances

Impotentia erigendi and impotentia coeundi are very unusual as initial symptoms (Sloof et al. 1964; Guidetti, Fortuna et al. 1964: a cervical astrocytoma with the patient unable to ejaculate, and with spastic paraparesis; Berciano et al. 1982). They are also unusual as the initial symptoms in conus medullaris tumours.

Subarachnoid haemorrhage

Subarachnoid haemorrhage secondary to a spinal tumour is a classic acquisition in neurosurgery but is a very rare event.
Considering the importance and the frequency of aneurismal and AVMs subarachnoid haemorrhage, we think it proper to dwell on this syndrome.

The first description is by André-Thomas et al. (1930) in a caudal tumour; later Abbott (1938) in a filum terminale ependymoma. Nasser and Correll (1968) collected only 15 cases and Djindjian et al. (1978) 45, reported in literature. More recently Vernet et al. (1986) report an exhaustive review of literature.

The patient feels a sharp dorsal or dorsolumbar pain (in cono-caudal tumours), without loss of consciousness.
A meningeal syndrome is established and associated, in cono-caudal gliomas, with cruralgia and sciatalgia; cerebrospinal fluid is blood-stained.
It can be spontaneous or caused by a trauma or strong exertion. More often present in cono-caudal ependymomas (Abbott 1939; Werteimer et al. 1950; Fincher 1951; Mendelson and More 1958; Amici and Borghi 1959; Rand and Rand 1960; Iob et al. 1980; Kulali 1989; Herb et al. 1990; Malbrain et al. 1994), it can also be present in neurinomas (Fortuna and La Torre 1967; Prieto and Cantu 1967; De Divitiis et al. 1985; Bruni et al. 1991), astrocytomas, hemangioblastomas (Kormos 1980; Cerejo et al. 1990), and meningeal sarcomas. In one case of caudal "lacunar meningoblastoma" in an 8-year-old boy (Roger et al. 1949) and in a 34-year-old man with cono-caudal angioblastic meningioma (autoptic report after a negative bilateral angiography) (Nassar and Correll 1968), the subarachnoid haemorrhage was present in two high-vascular, often haemorrhagic tumours. The tumour histology is of considerable importance here: the filum terminale ependymomas have a loose, high-vascular connectival texture, unlike dense and resistant connectival-capsulated ependymomas at other levels. The frequency at the conus and caudal levels also has another explanation: here the mechanical stresses are greater during neck and rachis movements, and indeed in 1 out of 3 cases the haemorrhage occurred during physical activity (Djindjian et al. 1978).

Neurogenic claudicatio intermittens

This is a typical symptom of medullary stress. It consists of weakness and hyposthenia in first one lower limb then the other, which reveals itself while walking and decreases after a few minutes rest; it starts again when walking is resumed. Functional restoration becomes subsequently incomplete and spastic paraparesis occurs. During the initial phase, neurologic examination is negative when the patient is at rest, while first hypertonia and increase of deep reflexes, then evident pyramidal signs are revealed when he is under stress. Sensitivity remains intact and sphincteric disturbances are rare at the beginning.

Although more frequent in lumbar canal stenosis (Verbiest 1976) and in the oblitering vasculopathy of the lower limbs, in 1943 Wyburn and Mason found it in 2 cases of low-medullary hemangioblastomas and in 7 vascular malformations.

It is due to a medullary ischemia by direct or indirect (in radiculo-medullary arteries involvement) compression of the anterior spinal artery: the haematic supply becomes insufficent to provide for increased metabolism during a long walk.

Transverse section syndrome

Vertebral angioma can reveal itself in this manner, at times following a trauma or a pregnancy (Arseni and Simionescu 1959; Fortuna and Guidetti 1961). Haemorrhagic tumours can also start with this syndrome (Abbott 1939; Wertheimer et al. 1950; Fincher 1951; Mendelson and More 1958; Amici and Borghi 1959; Rand and Rand 1960; Fortuna and La Torre 1967).

The early syndrome

The need to associate the first symptom with the subsequent one becomes clear when we consider that spinal tumours reveal themselves through pain in 70% of cases, and with paresthesia and hypoesthesia in 5-20%, complaints usually attributable to several diseases such as "arthritis", "neuritis" or " visceral diseases".

The second symptom is almost always diagnostically clearer and defines or contributes to determine an organic neurological syndrome with features of medullary, radicular or radiculo-medullary lesion.

Hence the utility of its study, for the most part absent in the literature, except for intramedullary gliomas, as we suggested in 1964 when pointing out that the second symptom was well remembered by patients because it was more serious.

In the same study we pointed out that the early syndrome was purely the result of the patient's own, and thus anamnestic, data. Neurological examination data are even more productive of useful diagnostic elements, as Sloof et al. (1964) state: an unusual initial pain already has a correspondence in reflex modifications.

More recently, with regard to intramedullary tumours, Cristofori et al. (1991) state that "a precocious diagnosis is hardly attainable in this pathology", but they also added that of the 113 patients operated on in 12 years (1979-1991), "only in the last 3 years have 11 patients reached the operating stage with an algic syndrome and negative neurological examination, and only 9% was studied with MRI".

In a careful study on spinal meningiomas, based on a wide review of existing literature, Pagni (1989) states that spinal meningioma is often operated on after a long clinical history.

The frequency, association and type of complaint vary according to the site of the tumour; it is thus essential to examine the early syndrome in relation to it.

Cervical tumours

More than 50% of cervical tumours are neurinomas and meningiomas, followed by intramedullary tumours (30%) and extradural malignancy (6-7%) (Webb et al. 1953).

The frequency of neurinomas compared with meningiomas is in some series almost double (25:15, Torma 1957; 88:43, Sloof et al. 1964), while in others it is almost the same (Broager 1953; Arseni and Ionesco 1958; Chigasachi and Pennibacher 1968; Iraci et al. 1971); or lower (Ectors et al. 1960; Scaglietti et al. 1971; Pagni 1989).

Neurinomas frequently arise from IV-V-VI root, while meningiomas above all affect the higher cervical segments (Webb et al. 1953); at the foramen magnum the meningiomas/neurinomas relation is 6:1 (Love et al. 1954; Dodge et al. 1956; Stein et al. 1963). In childhood and adolescence there is a greater incidence of glioma (in particular astrocytomas, seldom ependymomas) (Rand and Rand 1960).

The most schematic precocious syndrome is presented by neurinomas: a unilateral, monoradicular, persistent pain often occurring at night, increased by decubitus, followed after some time by various degrees of hypoesthesia or weakness at the same radicular level. This is almost pathognomonic in neurinomas, although it can be caused by lateral disk herniation, but in this last condition the pain is sharper and the onset and development of weakness faster.

More frequently *meningiomas* cause a short initial syndrome formed above all by paresthesia and radicular pain (Broager 1953; Torma 1957; Pagni 1989) and sometimes unilateral weakness, followed by precocious, motor and/or sensitive long-tract involvement.

The paresthesias at the distal end of the lower limb at times appear before paraparesis, which is always more serious in the homolateral limb.

In foramen magnum tumours, more often meningiomas than neurinomas, the initial complaints particularly affect the upper limbs.

In foramen magnum meningiomas and neurinomas the precocious syndrome is almost the same and is characterized by an often strong occipital pain, followed by paresthesias or paresis in one upper limb or both, in contrast with the rule whereby cervical neurinomas and meningiomas never, in the initial stage of the disease, affect the upper limbs (except for radicular deficiency), involving the homolateral lower limb and then the controlateral one.

In this precocious stage, beyond these syndromes characteristic of neurinoma or meningioma, and sometimes within their fields, the X-ray can frequently give the diagnosis: where an enlargement of a neural foramen occurs, this almost always indicates a neurinoma.

The onset of *extradural malignancy* is characterized by a sharp radicular pain (50% of cases), often pluriradicular, alone or with tenacious vertebral pain or radicular paresthesia. Mono- or bilateral weakness rapidly manifests itself, starting or immediately appearing as more serious in the lower limbs; it happens without any radiographic extradural malignancy features in the X-ray (Lindgren 1954; Torma 1957: 42.3% of 223 cases; Paillas et al. 1963); in this phase there may be an increase in the erythrocyte sedimentation rate. When, however, there exist osteolitic or osteoblastic phenomena, the X-ray (osteolysis of the one or more vertebral body or neural arches; destruction of one or both pedicles) allows the diagnosis of extradural malignancy of insidious onset, such as some carcinomas, primary osteogenic tumours, sarcomas or plasmocytomas.

In *intramedullary tumours* monoradicular pain, mono- or bilateral, is rare, both at the beginning and at the late stages of the disease; the pain is indicative only when it clearly possesses the features of cornual pain. Cordonal pain has an important diagnostic value when localized in the trunk and/or in the lower limbs, but rarely occurs. Actually, even without this pain, weakness is present in more than 70% of cases as primary or secondary symptom, and can have a great diagnostic value, since in most cases radicular paresis occurs, limited to the upper limbs (bilateral from the beginning or subsequently affecting the limbs), sometimes preceded by fasciculations and linked to paresthesias or to a mono- or bilateral segmental touch and temperature hypoesthesia. These disturbances are due to an involvement of the anterior and posterior horns and of the spinothalamic tract. In the astrocytomas and other gliomas in our cases the weakness arose earlier and was more frequent than in ependymomas.

Cervico-dorsal gliomas, those with simultaneous involvement of contiguous cervical and dorsal segments, can cause a precocious syndrome with different features from those of dorsal or cervical gliomas. Vertebral pain can simultaneously involve the nape and back. The weakness can be serious or moderate spastic mono- or paraparesis but associated with hypotrophy of the small hand muscles. This syndrome is usual in cervical spondylotic myelopathy, which can cause segmental hypoesthesia with vascular pathogenesis (Guidetti 1958), although here the pseudomyotonic phenomenon of hand opening, noticed in 47% of cases (Fortuna and Silipo 1961) is usual if not pathognomonic, and characterized by a remarkable slowness in the extension motion of the fist, especially in the 4th and 5th finger, while the closing was strong and fast. The weakness in the extension of the fingers has to be accompanied by a remarkable pyramidalization of the hand (Alemà 1958). This motor syndrome of small hand muscles can be caused by anterior midline meningiomas not infrequently with fasciculations (Austin 1960) and by some inferior cervical neurinomas (Arseni and Ionesco 1958). It is very frequent in meningiomas or neurinomas of the foramen magnum and is caused by involvement of the anterior spinal artery (Love et al. 1954; Dodge et al. 1956; Stein et al. 1963); muscle atrophy is combined with spastic tetraparesis, and only descending progression of a possible cordonal pain, from the upper limbs or trunk to the lower limbs, would suggest an intramedullary site.

Dorsal tumours

This region is the more frequent location for neoplastic compressions of the spinal cord.

The *neurinomas* are almost 40-51%, with a male preponderance (3:2) (Broager 1953; Torma 1957; Arseni and Ionesco 1958; Sloof et al. 1964; Iraci et al. 1971). In neurinomas radicular pain is the most frequent initial symptom, but diagnosis is made later than in cervical neurinoma both because the motor and sensitive radicular deficiencies that follow the pain are not so evident in the trunk as in the limbs, but above all because radicular pain can reproduce a visceral pain (Eeg-Olofsson et al. 1981).

In fact in most cases the precocious syndrome is marked by an initial monoradicular pain, mono- or bilateral, combined with motor long-tract signs. 70-85% of spinal *meningiomas* arises in the dorsal column (Elsberg 1941: 70%; Oddsson 1947: 83% of the 305 cases reviewed from the literature; Broager 1953: 83.7%; Guidetti and Carloni 1955: 77%; Torma 1957: 85%; Arseni and Ionesco 1958: 88%; Bernasconi and Cassinari 1961: 87%; Davis and Washburn 1970: 77%; Rupp 1970: 89%; Iraci et al. 1971: 73.4%; Scaglietti et al. 1971: 64%; Nittner 1976: 69.7%; Levy et al. 1982: 73%; Wen-Qing 1982: 69.5%; Pagni 1989 in the review of 1888 cases: 1486 cases = 78.5%, 68 cases dorsolumbar = 3.56%).

The female/male ratio is 4:1; in children too, the only two meningiomas occurred in girls (Rand and Rand 1960). In dorsal meningiomas the initial stage is mono- and oligosymptomatic, with radicular and vertebral pain, sometimes combined with long-tract sensory or motor deficiency, above all paresthesias at the distal end of the lower limbs. Medullary compression can later cause a Brown-Séquard syndrome (mostly spurious and incomplete), or a paraparesis, more serious in the homolateral limb, and a superficial sensory deficiency with ascending development. Brown-Séquard syndrome can also be present at cervical level, but is more frequent at the dorsal segment.

In our cases of cervical compression, this syndrome was more frequent in spondylogenetic myelopathy and always much less atypical than in tumoral compressions, often for the lack of one clinical aspect (Fortuna and Giuffrè 1962).

The Brown-Séquard syndrome, extremely indicative of extramedullary compression – Arseni and Ionesco 1958: neurinomas: 12.6% (12/95), meningiomas: 7% (8/114), intramedullary tumours: 6.8% (5/73, of which 69 gliomas) – has rarely been verified in the initial stage of the disease.

Extradural malignancies have a high incidence (60%), especially those with metastasis (Torma 1957). In childhood, primitive tumours are more frequent: sarcomas usually in children around the age of 10 and sympatoblastomas (neuroblastomas) in those aged 0-3 (Laubicher 1967; Chodkiewiez et al. 1970). The Brown-Séquard syndrome does not always correspond to that reported for cervical localization: severe vertebral pains (60%), but also radicular (24%), at times combined;

subacute evolution of medullary compression with sensory and motor deficiency, distal at first, and moderate increase of the ESR.

Radicular pain, especially pluriradicular, is severe, often bilateral, "belt-like", and has great diagnostic value. The evolution is faster than in cervical compressions on account not only of the narrowness of the dorsal canal, but above all of the high rate of the metastases (69%), which have a faster evolution than primary tumours, and for the greater vulnerability of dorsal cord circulation. The onset of weakness in the lower limbs in most cases not only manifests itself abruptly but, contrary to cervical localizations, rapidly evolves into paraplegia, although rare, apoplectic onset and rapid evolution have also been noted in other spinal tumours (gliomas: Sloof et al. 1964; Guidetti, Fortuna et al. 1964).

The dorsal and lumbosacral *gliomas* have a different frequency (Sloof et al. 1964: 58.7%; Guidetti and Fortuna 1975: 39.9%); among intramedullary tumours the probabilities of an ependymoma seem to be very low at every age when the duration of the clinical history is less than a year (Sloof et al. 1964; Guidetti, Fortuna et al. 1964); in most dorsal gliomas the early syndrome is characterized by a frequently painful mono- or paraparesis more often cordonal or vertebral than radicular, with or without sensory impairment, and rarely with sphincteric disturbances. We have to stress that, in our gliomas, a motor impairment, unilateral at first, has never become bilateral during the precocious stage of the disease. When it was bilateral, it arose or developed with this feature.

At a precocious stage, an initial radicular pain thus suggests a neurinoma; more rarely it indicates a meningioma, and sporadically a glioma.

A frequent clinical aspect in the precocious stage of dorsal gliomas is cordonal pain localized in the thorax and abdomen with descending evolution; the most important and constant sign is segmental hypo-anesthesia. Unlike the cervical and dorsolumbar regions, the high and middle dorsal segments do not innervate relevant muscles, so deficiency and hypotrophies of the dorsal and intercostal muscles are rarely recognized or visible. Dorsal fasciculations can be observed.

The Brown-Séquard syndrome has been also noticed in intramedullary tumours, but we are unable to say whether at a precocious stage. In 1916 Karger reported a typical case and quoted Malise, that referred there were only two known cases at that time. Cases like these are also reported by Elsberg (1925), Kernhoan et al. (1931) and Jerasek (1932). In the Guidetti and Fortuna's cases (1964) (46 gliomas) the incidence was 6.5% (2 cervical and 1 dorsal), and always atypical.

The lumbosacral gliomas often begin with radicular pain, and in most cases are mistaken for sciatalgia secondary to disk herniation (Guidetti and Fortuna 1975: 83%).

Tumoral sciatalgia is difficult to interpret when no other complaints are in evidence (Love 1944; Fortuna et al. 1970; Wiss 1982). The intermittent pain, typical of disc herniation, is often observed in oncogenic sciatalgias (Love 1944; Fortuna et al. 1970: 50%). Exacerbation of pain at night, together with a negative result of the straight-leg-raising test are the most indicative signs of a spinal tumour. As mentioned above, neoplastic sciatalgias are always attributed to disc herniation, the misunderstanding stemming from epidemiological criteria: the incidence of disc herniation is very much higher than spinal tumours.

In the lumbosacral gliomas the sciatic pain is not so clear as in neurinomas and often involves cornual pain, which is lacerating and burning; it can last a considerable time as an initial symptom, and can suggest a tumour when there are irregularly-distributed indications that the upper and lower motor neuron is affected, i.e. spastic and flaccid weakness, sometimes with fasciculations and irregular hypoesthesia.

In conclusion, in most cases the precocious syndrome is characterized by radicular pain, sciatalgia in particular, mono- or bilateral combined with flaccid mono- or paraparesis often not corresponding: unilateral sciatica with paraparesis, or the contrary, monoparesis with bilateral radicular pain.

Very rarely paresthesia and hypoesthesia are associated with it; these are more often independent of motor deficiency and can be associated with sphincteric disorders; as at the cervical level, a unilateral motor deficiency can become bilateral during the evolution of the early syndrome.

Cono-filum tumours

Given that the spinal canal at the lumbosacral level is very wide, that the lumbar enlargement corresponds to D_{10}-D_{11}-D_{12}-L_1 and that under L_1 there are lumbar, sacral and coccygeal roots (cauda equina), a small D_{12}-L_1 tumour can affect a number of neuromeres and even more roots. Moreover, a caudal tumour can reach a remarkable size before clinical manifestations arise. If the compression is at the epiconus or caudal level, the impairment will be different, spastic paraparesis and sensory deficiency with a level, and flaccid paresis with sensory radicular deficiency respectively.

Meningioma. Lumbar meningiomas are rare. The radicular pain is often the first symptom and, when exacerbated by column motion or decubitus, can be long-lasting. It can spread as sciatica, mono- or, rarely, bilateral, the vertebral pain indicating the segment of one of the affected roots.

Sensory deficiency. "Saddle" and perianal or genital hypo-anesthesia are the main sensory deficiency provoked by tumours affecting the 3rd, 4th, 5th sacral root or the corresponding neuromeres.

Motor deficiency. Spastic or flaccid paresis or paralisis can be observed. In the precocious stages fasciculations without evident atrophies can be observed but weakness and hypotonia are already present; the preservation of anal and bulbo-cavernous reflex means integrity of the conus.

Sexual and sphincteric disorders. When the conus is involved, urgent micturition and incontinence are precocious. Later on constipation and fecal incontinence become evident. There are no clinically differential elements between lumbosacral neurinoma and meningioma and the filum terminalis ependymoma. The only different feature may be sensory deficiency: "saddle" in meningiomas and neurinomas, while in the lower limbs in ependymomas.

Neurinoma. Neurinoma can begin with sciatalgia (while it is rare in meningiomas), although it is more frequently associated with either a spastic-flaccid motor deficiency, or a radicular-cordonal sensory deficiency with regular distribution (while in gliomas it is irregular). This also occurs when the initial disturbance is abdomino-inguinal neuralgia or lumbocruralgia; it is more frequent in neurinomas but not uncommon in gliomas. X-ray rarely helps in the diagnosis of dorsal or lumbosacral medullary compressions because the increase of interpeduncular distance or an enlargement of a neural foramen is unlikely. These radiological signs are difficult to interpret, as indeed is any pedicle erosion present; only calcification suggests a meningioma, but they are rare even at an advanced stage.

Extradural malignancy. These tumours can start with serious vertebral pains, often combined with violent and wide-spread radicular ones in the lower limbs. These pains are rapidly followed by serious mono- or bilateral flaccid and spastic-flaccid motor deficiency. The beginning can also consist of paraparesis, distal at first, with concomitant or rapidly subsequent sensory deficiency. The tumours mainly prove to be metastatic, as at the dorsal and dorsolumbar level, or, less frequently, sarcomatous.

Pathological anatomy

Spinal tumours can be divided into intra- and extradural; intradural can be intra- and extramedullary.

Intradural extramedullary tumours

In most cases these consist of meningiomas, neurinomas and neurofibromas. Dysembryogenetic tumours (dermoid, epidermoid and neurenteric cysts), or malignant neoplasias (metastasis of haematic and CSF origin) are rare.

Meningioma. This is a benign tumour with a clear predominance in women, with its greatest incidence between the 5th and 7th decade. It forms nearly 25% of spinal tumours and nearly 13% of all meningiomas. Spinal meningioma is more frequent at the dorsal segment while the lumbar same is very rare. The tumour consists of a firm, well demarcated, reddish-brown mass, more frequently anterolateral to the spinal cord. Dural attachment of the lesion is always present; like intracranial meningiomas, this originates in the arachnoid cells. Although all types of meningioma may be present (syncytial, transitional, fibroblastic, angioblastic and sarcomatous), the most common at the spinal level is the transitional, psammomatous meningioma.

Neurinoma. Together with neurofibroma, this constitutes 25-30% of intradural extramedullary tumours. The neurinoma, or schwannoma, consists of an encapsulated, ovalar, lobulated, whitish mass. The radicular structures appear eccentric to the mass, running into the tumour capsule. Histologically it is formed by interwoven bundles of spindle cells (Type A of Antoni) or by a looser, mixoid texture (Type B of Antoni).

Neurofibroma. Frequently observed in von Recklinghausen's neurofibromatosis, this has a firmer texture than neurinoma, less clear demarcation, and cannot be dissected from the roots that run through the tumour. Microscopically it is composed of Schwann's cells, fibroblasts and collagen fibres intermingled in a mucoid or mixoid matrix.

Dermoid cysts. These constitute 0.5-1% of spinal tumours, but reach 10% in childhood. Congenital lesions which come from epithelial inclusion of the neural crest between the 3rd and 5th week, they more frequently develop in the lumbar segment. Muscle-scheletric anomalies such as spina bifida or dermal sinus are frequently present. They appear as different-sized, well-demarcated, opaque, ovalar masses. The cut surface reveals a yellowish, butter-like material due to secretion of sebaceous glands, hair follicles and sudoriferous glands.

Epidermoid cysts. Epidermoid cysts are rarer than dermoid ones. Macroscopically they appear as small pearly masses with butter-like content, rich in cholesterin, the result of the desquamation of malpidian epithelium.

Extradural tumours

These derive from osteo-legamentous and condroid structures of the column, with subsequent involvement of the nervous structures.

Benign bone tumours
Osteoid osteoma. These constitute nearly 12% of primitive bone tumours in all sites, and 6% of spinal bone tumours. They appear as a small brownish mass, 1-2 cm in diameter, well-demarcated, surrounded by an osteosclerotic edge. Histologically they are composed of osteblastic aggregates surrounded by fibrovascular tissue.

Osteoblastoma. Rarer than osteomas osteoid, these represent nearly 1% of bone tumours. They are classified together with osteoid osteomas, the difference between them being represented by the size of the lesion: lesions under 2 cm in diameter are defined as osteoid osteomas, while bigger tumours are osteoblastomas. Histologically they are similar even if malignant degenerations are commoner in osteoblastomas.

Giant-cell tumours. Giant-cell tumours account for nearly 5% of primitive bone tumours and the incidence in the vertebral column is of 2-5%. There is a slight predominance in women, its greater incidence occurring roughly in the 3rd decade. More frequent at the sacral level, and in most cases involving the vertebral body, it consists of an osteolitic lesion formed by multinucleate giant cells and by reactive cells in the highly-vascularized matrix. Haemorrhages are also present.

Malignant bone tumours
Osteosarcoma. After metastatic lesions, these are the most common malignant bone tumours. They affect fast-growing bones and so are more easily noticed in long bone metaphysis or in pathological conditions of fast bone rearrangement such as Paget's disease or during radiation therapy. They are commonly associated with bilateral retinoblastoma. Macroscopically they appear as a highly-vascularized mass composed of an osseous neoformation in various phases of calcification. Microscopically they are composed of pathological bone tissue organized in little masses with a highly-vascularized stroma. Such bone neoformations are surrounded by neoplastic osteoblasts which assume the aspect of spindle or polygonal cells with frequent atypical mitosis. These atypical cells can also produce a non-osseous tissue: the osteosarcoma is classified thus into osteogenic, chondrogenic and fibrogenic osteosarcoma.

Ewing's sarcoma. At spinal level they are very rare, constituting 0.5% of malignant bone tumours of the column, with a definite predominance in men above all during the first two decades. Macroscopically they appear as a white-greyish, friable, often very vascularized mass, with sometimes spontaneous bleeding. Histologically they appear as a tumour with a predominant cellular component formed by small cells bundles. They are round with scarce and pale cytoplasma and ovalar nuclei. Mitoses are rare. Often present are necrosis areas with still living cells, which assume a pseudorosette aspect. The neoplastic cells spread throughout the osseous trabeculae and affect the cortical vascular channels and the periosteum.

Cartilaginous tumours
Osteochondroma. Although a rather frequent bone tumour (8-9% of all bone tumours), this is rare at the spinal level (1-4%). It is benign and generally solitary but in 10% of cases is multiple. Macroscopically it consists of a small exostotic mass arising from spinous apophyses or from transverse processes, formed by bone cortical covered by chondroid tissue. The cortical is in touch with spongy bone, in continuity with the vertebral same. All osteochondroma tissues are cytologically normal, with neoplastic degeneration in nearly 1% of the cases regarding a solitary osteochondroma, in nearly 10-15% if multiple.

Chondrosarcoma. This is a malignant tumour which forms in chondroid tissue both as a degeneration of a benign cartilaginous tumour (secondary chondrosarcoma) in 15% of cases, and as a primitively malignant one in 85%. The presence of the hyaline cartilage gives the tumour the aspect of an opalescent, irregular mass of variable dimensions. Histologically it is composed of anaplastic and often binucleate chondrocytes, with necrosis and cellular pleomorphism. It is divided into 3 types according to the degree of malignancy, the third being more anaplastic and biologically malignant.

Lipoma. This is classified among the congenital malformations of spinal occult dysraphism and is associated with meningocele, dermic sinus and tethered cord. In relation to such dysraphic states, it is usually of both intra- and extradural localization, mainly at cauda equina level. It is composed of normal fat cells, which, in extradural cases, are in direct continuity with the adipose subcutaneous tissue.

Angiolipoma. A benign tumour which forms 0.1-1.2% of spinal tumours, this is more commonly extradural, even if some sporadic intramedullary cases have been reported. The dorsal tract of the column is the most frequently affected. It is composed of mature fat cells and of pathological vessels with arteriolar and venular aspects, similar to arteriovenous malformations.

Chordoma. Since its description in 1857, about 1,000 cases have been reported in literature. Forming about 18% of malignant bone tumours, it has an ectodermic (notochordal) origin, thus generally involving the axial skeleton, but is unusual at dorsal level. Non-axial chordomas (involving for example a transverse process or a scapula) are very rare and of unclear origin.
In spite of its embryologic origin, the tumour does not, in spinal chordoma, appear in the nucleus pulposus but in the vertebral body, probably as a result of notochordal tissue at this level. Macroscopically it appears as a bulky, soft, gelatinous, invasive but not infiltrative

mass. Histologically it is composed of cells known as physaliphorous ("soap bubble") with a wide vacuolate cytoplasm, and inserted into a mucoid stroma. Two histological types are reported: typic and chondroid, with a better prognosis for the latter (4.1 years of life-expectancy for the classic type versus 15.8 years for the chondroid).

Vascular bone tumours

Vertebral angioma. While not rare (10-12% in autoptic series) this can be symptomatic in about 1% of cases with a clear predominance in women. It is a slow growing tumour composed of pathological vessels characterized by endothelial cells spread into a stroma formed by bone trabeculae and fat tissue.

Aneurysmatic bone cyst. This consists of a high-vascularized, multiloculated, osteolitic lesion often containing degraded haematic products, and is formed histologically of bloody cavities, without endothelium, and a basal lamina. The solid parts are formed of spindled cells immersed in a collagen stroma with frequent reactive giant cells.

Spinal metastases

These are the commonest malignant lesions of the column, autoptic series revealing vertebral metastases in 15-40% of patients who died from disseminated neoplasms. All vertebral bodies can be affected, although the low dorsal and lumbar tracts are more frequently involved. In the adult, metastases from lung, breast and prostatic carcinomas are frequent together with haemolymphopoietic tumours such as lymphomas and multiple myelomas. Metastasis from renal carcinoma and melanoma are also reported. In children extradural metastases are very rare and arise from Ewing's sarcoma, neuroblastoma, Hodgkin's disease, soft tissue sarcomas or germinal cell tumours. Although primitive epidural metastases are possible, the epidural space with relative medullary compression is subsequently affected by a primitive metastasis of the vertebral body.

Intramedullary tumours

These derive mainly from glial medullary cells and vascular structures, and are rarely metastatic lesions.

Glial tumours. These are ependymomas, astrocytomas, and rarely glioblastoma multiforme.
Ependymoma. This constitutes 4-6% of CNS tumours, about 1/3 of which affects the spinal cord, representing the most frequent intramedullary tumour in adults.
Macroscopically the spinal cord appears enlarged, the vessels stretched and distended. The tumour appears frequently demarcated, with a well-defined cleavage plane, and intra- or peri-tumoral cysts are usually present. Histologically they are benign, and originate from ependyma cells, mostly in the posterior part of the spinal cord, among the posterior cords, and can affect a number of medullary metameres. They can be totally removed. Some originate from the filum terminale or cono-filum causing a cono-caudal compression syndrome.

Astrocytoma. In adulthood these represent 30-40% of intramedullary tumours, and about 70% in childhood. The spinal cord is affected by macroscopic morphologic modifications similar to ependymoma, except the delimitation of the surrounding parenchyma which appears fully infiltrated by the tumour, and without a clear-cut cleavage plane. This makes the total removal of the mass possible if not easy. Histologically they are usually fibrillary astrocytomas.

Glioblastoma multiforme. The spinal glioblastoma multiforme is quite rare and forms 0.2-1.5% of intramedullary tumours, the literature reporting some 200 cases. It is infiltrative, friable, variegated and histologically characterized by a remarkable cellular polymorphism, with necrosis and vascular proliferation areas with frequent atypical mitosis.

Vascular structure tumours

Hemangioblastoma. Forming 1.5% of intramedullary tumours, this is spheroid, highly-vascularized, and often cystic. Histologically it is composed of thin-walled, strictly-interwoven blood vessels, and spreads in a stroma formed by large, pale cells. It can be totally removed.

Spinal cavernous angioma. Before MRI this was considered an exceptional occurrence at spinal level. At present the diagnosis of spinal cavernoma still only accounts for some 0.1-0.5% of spinal tumours. Its macroscopic and histological aspect is similar to that of cerebral cavernoma. The tumour appears as a small reddish-brown mass, composed of strictly interwoven blood vessels with neither stroma nor glial tissue in their context. Small haemorrhages are frequent. It can be totally removed.

Intramedullary metastases

These are very rare and can be haematic or CSF in origin. The former type consists of lung metastatic carcinoma or haemo-lymphopoietic neoplasms, while the latter is represented by neoplastic seeding of cerebral tumours such as medulloblastomas, pineal tumours and intraventricular ependymomas.

Radiological diagnosis

It is common knowledge that at present the radiological diagnosis of spinal tumours is based on computerized images (CT, MRI). Today myelography is used only for CT with intrarachidial contrast medium. The greater utility of CT or MRI in the specific case will depend on the characteristics and relations of the tumour. MRI, however, is clearly better than CT in the localization and anatomical definition of intramedullary tumours, cavernous angiomas and AVM. One of the limits of CT, connected with its method of image formation, consists of the need to discover the spinal segment to investigate using other diagnostic tools (clinical, neurophysiological, or radiological), while with MRI it is possible to effect "panoramic", multiplanar scans of the whole CNS. From a surgical point of view it is extremely important, because the surgeon has to know in advance and with certainty the site, extention and, possibly, nature of the tumour.

We shall now examine the radiological features of spinal tumours in relation to their position: intradural extramedullary, extradural, and intramedullary tumours.

Intradural extramedullary tumours

These are mainly meningiomas and neurinomas; malignant tumours are very rare, and are above all metastases of intracranial lesions such as medulloblastomas or ependymoblastomas spread through the CSF (neoplastic seeding). It is possible to find congenital malformations such as AVM, arachnoid or neuroenteric cysts.

Neurinomas. These are clearly evidenced both by CT and MRI. The non-enhanced TC (NETC) reveals both secondary osseous alteration as pedicle erosion with widening of intervertebral foramina or scalloping of the posterior part of the vertebral body, and an iso- or slightly hyperdense lesion with clear enhancement after i.v. contrast material. In bigger tumours, even if intradural extramedullary in origin, the greater development is extradural with invasion of paravertebral soft tissues, through a worn or destroyed intervertebral foramen. There may be cystic aspects which appear hypodense. However, in cases in which the tumours are inside the spinal canal, and derive from Schwann's sheath of the posterior roots, an erosion of the intervertebral foramina is present. This origin explains the site of the tumour which, if small, is lateral or posterolateral to the spinal cord, with medullary contralateral dislocation and homolateral widening of the subarachnoid space, clearly revealed by myelo-CT.

The T1-weighted MR images show the neurinomas as an hypointense lesion compared with the spinal cord in nearly 80% of cases, and isointense in 20% (Fig. 1) (Matsumoto et al. 1993). The limits are clear in the majority of cases, and a narrow contact area with the dura is present. Enhancement by paramagnetic contrast medium is notable in almost all cases (Figs. 2-3-4), and dishomogeneous or ring shaped in 60% (Matsumoto et al. 1993). In T2-weighted images, the lesion is hyperintense in nearly 80% of cases (Ishii et al. 1991; Hu et al. 1992; Li et al. 1992) and isointense in 20% (Matsumoto et al. 1993) In T2 and contrast-enhanced T1-weighted images there could be a "target image", with a hyperintense margin and hypointense core, possible the expression of cystic evolution (Sakai et al. 1992; Varma et al. 1992).

Meningiomas. The NECT shows an iso- or slightly hyperdense lesion with a light i.v. contrast enhancement. Pedicles erosions are usually absent and, in 3% of ca-

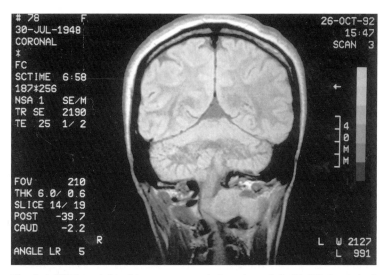

Fig. 1. MRI T1-weighted image; coronal view: large left C1-C2 dumb-bell (intra-extraforaminal) isointense tumour; late diagnosis. Histology: neurinoma.

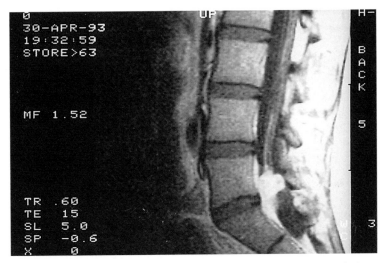

Fig. 2. MRI gadolinium-enhanced T1-weighted image; sagittal view: highly hyperintense small tumour at the level of the cauda equina. Histology: neurinoma.

ses, there are intra-tumoral calcifications, clearly evidenced by CT (Solero et al. 1989; Osborn 1994). The tumour is seldom massively calcified (Lunardi et al. 1992).

MRI evidences the tumour clearly, revealing it in almost 80% of cases as iso-hypointense compared with the cord in T1-weighted images (Fig. 5), and as hyper-

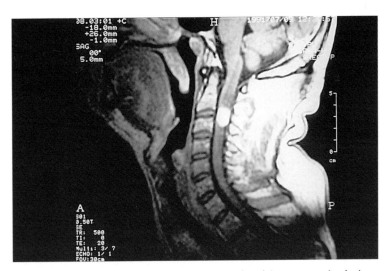

Fig. 3. MRI gadolinium-enhanced T1-weighted image; sagittal view: roundish hyperintense anterolateral tumour at C2-C3-level. Histology: neurofibroma.

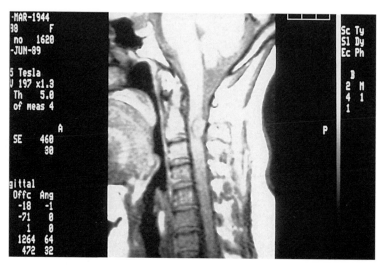

Fig. 4a. MRI gadolinium-enhanced T1-weighted image; sagittal view: hyperintense lesion at the C2-C3 level. Histology: neurinoma.

intense in nearly 20%. In nearly 75% of cases it is iso-hypointense in T2-weighted images (Fig. 6) (Solero et al. 1989; Matsumoto et al. 1993).

A more frequent hyperintensity in T2-weighted image is reported in syncitial and angioblastic meningiomas. The tumour edges can be lobulated and dural insertion is usually large (Matsumoto et al. 1993). An homogeneous, usually unpronounced contrast enhancement is present. In completely calcified cases it appears hypointense in all sequences, with scarce contrast-enhancement (Chaparro et al. 1992; Osborn 1994).

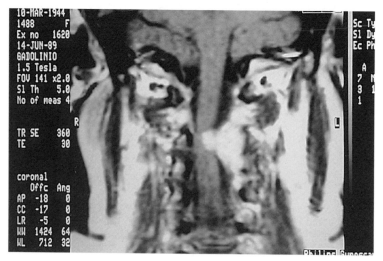

Fig. 4b. MRI gadolinium-enhanced T1-weighted image; coronal view: left posterolateral hyperintense dumb-bell tumour. Histology: neurinoma.

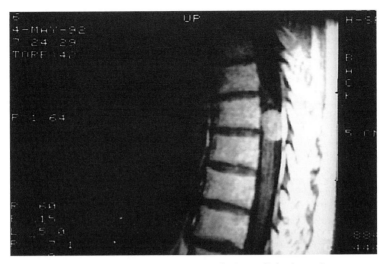

Fig. 5a. MRI T1-weighted image; sagittal view: slight hyperintense posterolateral tumour at T7-T8 level. Histology: meningioma.

Even if T1 and T2 signal characteristics are generally alike in meningiomas and
neurinomas (Matsumoto et al. 1993; Osborn 1994) other MRI parameters can be
useful for differential diagnosis. They are mainly represented by tumour margins,
which are more regular in neurinomas, and sometimes lobulated in meningiomas;
by dural insertion, definitely larger in meningiomas with possible evidencing of
"dural tail" (hyperintense appearance of dural peri-tumoral structures) (Lunardi et
al. 1993; Matsumoto et al. 1993; Osborn 1994); by gadolinium-enhancement

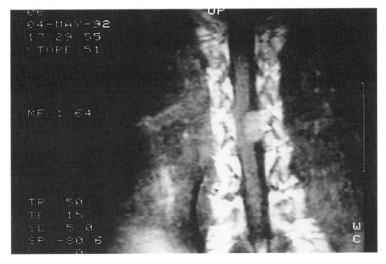

Fig. 5b. MRI T1-weighted image; coronal view: slight hyperintense posterolateral tumour at T7-T8 level. Histology: meningioma.

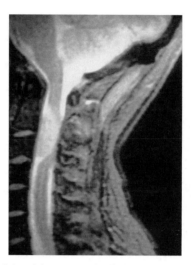

Fig. 6. MRI T2-weighted image; sagittal view: irregularly iso-hyperintense tumour at C2-C3 level with noticeable spinal cord posterior dislocation. Histology: meningioma.

modalities, more marked and at times irregular in neurinomas, while slight and homogeneous in meningiomas (this last aspect seems to be due to ultrastructural differences in "gap-junctions", more sinusoidal, tortuous, and extended in meningiomas than in neurinomas (Long et al. 1973; Watabe et al. 1989; Matsumoto et al. 1993).

Dermoid cysts. These can be congenital or acquired. The former are dysembriogenetic in origin, while the latter are almost always iatrogenic (consequences of lumbar tap by which epidermic elements can be implanted in the subarachnoid space (Choremis et al. 1958; Kudo et al. 1980). Congenital cysts are often associated with spinal dysraphism such as spina bifida or hemivertebrae. The CT shows them as hypodense masses while the MRI is variable but more frequently iso-hyperintense in comparison with CSF in all sequences (Fig. 7) (Osborn 1994).

Intradural metastasis. With MRI the diagnosis of intradural metastasis has become more frequent (Schunecht 1992). More often these metastases are from medulloblastomas or ependymomas, even if they are also apparent in pineoblastomas, in multiform glioblastomas and from carcinomas of the plexus choroideus. They spread through liquoral neoplastic seeding. Non-enhanced MRI seldom provides useful information, given the small dimensions of metastases and of the isointensity signal in relation to the spinal cord. They are well evidenced by i.v. contrast enhancement: even small tumours are clearly enhanced and are easily identified with T1-weighted images. The CT and MRI are not specific, but the clinical picture will provide the necessary data for a correct diagnosis.

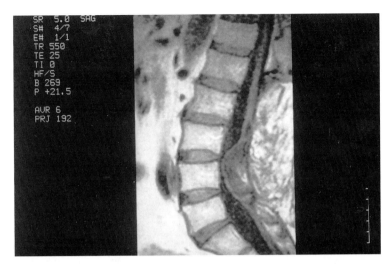

Fig. 7. MRI T1-weighted image; sagittal view: irregular roundish isointense mass, with an internal hyperintense core, at the level of the posterior aspect of the low lumbar canal. Histology: dermoid cyst.

Some cases of haematogenous spinal leptomeningeal metastases are also reported. The non-enhanced T1-weighted images fail to reveal such lesions, while the gadolinium-enhanced T1-weighted images show a thin, linear enhancement at the margin of the cord affecting either a few metameres or the whole cord (Lim et al. 1990).

Histologically the lesions are mostly melanomas, prostate, lung and breast carcinomas, and haemolymphopoietic neoplasms. Intramedullary metastases or the primitive intramedullary localizations of haemolymphopoietic neoplasms are very rare. In six cases radiologically described and observed pre-MRI, only a broadening of the spinal cord is reported (Hautzer et al. 1983).

Extradural tumours

These are mostly bone tumours, which then affect the epidural space with possible myeloradicular compression. Because of the relative protonic immobility of the mineralized bone matrix, the MRI presents less capability of determining cortical integrity and the tumour mineralization pattern than CT, while it is more useful for detecting the neoplastic involvement of the bone marrow, the intratecal development of the mass with possible myeloradicular compression, and the paravertebral spreading of the tumour.

Vertebral angioma. Typical in this tumour is the "corduroy cloth" appearance of the vertebral body showed by X-ray (Dorwart et al. 1983), an aspect evident only if 1/3 of the vertebral body is affected (Healy et al. 1983; Foxet al. 1993). CT is the optimal procedure to evaluate a pathology of the kind (Laredo et al. 1989; Nguyen et al. 1987). The analogous CT of the "corduroy cloth" aspect of the X-ray consists of evidencing a spotted vertebral body, determined by axial cutting of residual bone hypertrophic trabeculae in the fatty matrix crossed by pathological vessels (Ross et al. 1987). If the hypodense component of this mixed aspect, the sign of a greater fatty texture, is prevalent, it is probably a symptomatic evolution of the lesion (Laredo et al. 1989). A pathologic paravertebral tissue (usually neo-plastic extension or haematoma) may be present (Baker et al. 1986; Dagi et al. 1990). CT is also used for a biopsy of the lesion in order to differentiate possible metastatic lesions in doubtful cases (Gaston et al.1989; Nguyen et al. 1989).

The MRI aspect is, like that of CT, mixed with fatty tissue hyperintense in T1-weighted images, the hypertrophic trabeculae hypointense, with flow void areas in relation to the rich pathological vascularization (Fox et al. 1993).

MRI too can have a prognostic value: the mixed aspect described is in fact in-dicative of a non-evolutive and clinically silent lesion, while a more homoge-neously iso- or hypo-intense aspect is more frequent in the lesion's extraosseous extensions and in medullary compressions (Laredo et al. 1989). The lesion shows an evident gadolinium contrast-enhancement and no differential aspects in the en-hancement pattern of the lesion's evolution are reported (Fox et al. 1993).

Osteoid osteoma. This more frequently affects the pedicles or laminae, above all at the lumbar segment. It rarely compresses the nervous structures, revealing itself by radicular pains or metameric deficiencies (Dahilin et al. 1967; Sim et al. 1977). Osteoid osteoma with CT appears as a small, oval, hypodense area containing va-riable amounts of calcifications, sometimes surrounded by reactive hyperostosis. Contrast enhancement is present.

In the MRI the lesion appears hypo-isointense in T1-weighted images and hyper-intense in T2-weighted ones. Intra-tumoral calcification and marginal hyperosto-sis can provoke "target" images with an hypointense core (intra-tumoral calcifi-cation), an iso-hyperintense intermediate area (noncalcific neoplastic part), and a marginal hypointense marginal area (reactive osteosclerosis). A slight gadolinium enhancement is present (Osborne 1994).

Osteoblastoma. This is classified among osseous tumours together with osteoid os-teoma in comparison with which, however, it is bigger and sometimes more aggres-sive (Syklawer et al. 1990; Osborne 1994). The dorsal and lumbar segments are more frequently involved, in nearly 35% respectively (Sypert et al. 1990). It almost exclusively affects the posterior elements of the vertebra, subsequently affecting the vertebral body (Rossner et al. 1985; Azouz et al. 1986), an eventuality which, however, is very rare. In almost 50% of cases the lesion appears hypodense with CT, while in the remaining cases the lesions can be variegated, hyper- or hypo-

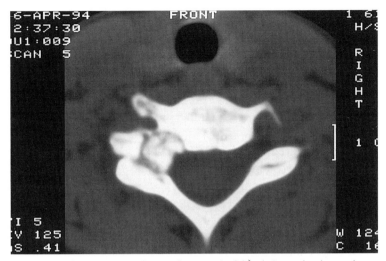

Fig. 8. Baseline CT scan focused at cervical level: irregular hyperdense mass disrupting the osseous border of the left lateral recess. Histology: osteoblastoma.

dense depending on the degree of tumoral calcifications (Nemoto et al. 1990) (Figs. 8-9); the edges are quite clear, with signs of hyperostosis and osteosclerosis in their relevant context (Dorwart 1983; Syklawer 1990).

The MRI, scantily reported in this lesion (Syklawer et al. 1990), reveals a mass which is mainly iso-hypointense in T1-weighted images and hyperintense in T2, with dishomogeneous gadolinium contrast enhancement. The peri-tumoral os-

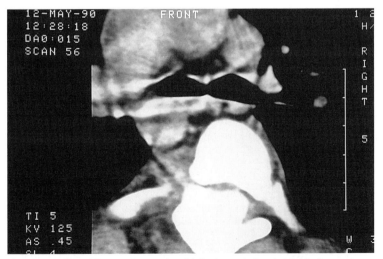

Fig. 9. Baseline CT scan focused at high thoracic level: highly hyperdense irregular mass occupying over than 80% of the vertebral canal, arising from the left posterolateral aspect of the vertebra. Histology: osteoblastoma.

teosclerotic area appears considerably hypointense in all sequences (Syklawer et al. 1990).

Osteosarcoma. In nearly 90% of cases this affects the vertebral body (Sundaresan et al. 1990). The CT shows an unclearly marginated lesion of mixed density because of osteolitic and calcificated areas. This exam points out possible intra- and extraspinal growths (De Santos et al. 1969; Bacci et al. 1982).
The MRI aspect depends on the calcification degree of the mass: more frequently there is a dishomogeneous lesion in T1-weighted images, and hyperintense in T2. However in less calcified tumours a hypo-isointense aspect predominates in T1-weighted images and hyperintense in T2, while more calcified tumours are hypointense in all sequences. The MRI is more sensitive than CT in detecting and quantifying intraspinal and paravertebral localizations, mainly because it provides multiplanar images (Osborn 1994).

Chordoma. The CT shows the lesion as a mainly hypodense area with hyperdense calcifications in almost 30-50% of cases (Dorwart et al. 1983; Yuh et al. 1988). It clearly evidences the neoplastic extraspinal part of the tumour, which is often bigger than its osseous counterpart, and is little enhanced by the contrast medium (Krol et al. 1983).
With RMI there is a dishomogeneous hypointensity in T1-weighted images and a marked hyperintensity in T2, in relation to a large amount of tumorous mucoid substance (Yuh et al. 1988). It is possible to distinguish the chondroid type, more hypointense both in T1 and T2-weighted images, in relation to the classic type (Sze et al. 1988; Sebag et al. 1993).

Giant-cell tumours. CT usually shows a hypodense area, sometimes with a hyperdense edge (osteosclerotic), while inside an iso-hypointense area in T1-weighted images and an iso-hyperintense area in T2 (Aoki et al. 1991), MRI may reveal haemosiderin deriving from previous small-scale bleeding of sinusoidal capillaries, more often present in mechanically-stressed osseous segments such as vertebrae, or the osseous segments of lower limbs, which appear hypointense both in T1 and T2-weighted images on account of haemosiderin (Aoki et al. 1991; Osborn et al. 1994).

Metastatic tumours. Spinal metastases, often multiple, are more frequent at low dorsal and lumbar level. They particularly affect the vertebral bodies, with subsequent growth in the extradural space and in the paravertebral soft tissues. They can be osteolytic, osteoblastic or mixed. The TC shows the substitution of thin osseous trabeculae of the vertebral bodies with pathological tissue and the possible cortical destruction with intraspinal and paravertebral spreading. Such tissue will be hyperdense in osteoblastic metastases and hypodense in osteolitic ones. With MRI

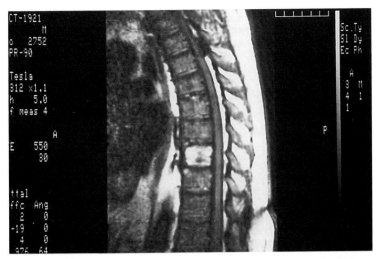

Fig. 10. MRI gadolinium-enhanced T1-weighted image; sagittal view: unhomogeneously hyperintense T9 lesion. Histology: osteolitic metastasis.

the bone marrow appears replaced by neoplastic tissue which, in osteolitic metastases, assumes an aspect which is dishomogeneously hypointense in T1-weighted images with gadolinium enhancement (Fig. 10) and hyperintense in T2. This aspect can be useful in the differential diagnosis between the "benign" pathological vertebral fracture (e.g. osteoporosis) and the "malignant" one (vertebral metastasis): in the former the bone marrow appears hyperintense in T1-weighted images, and hypointense in T2, while in the latter it is hypointense in T1 and hyperintense

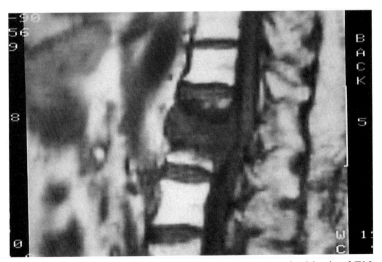

Fig. 11. MRI T1-weighted image; sagittal view: the vertebral body of T10 appears unhomogeneously hypointense. Histology: osteoblastic metastasis.

in T2 (Baker 1990; Osborn 1994). In osteoblastic lesions, the tumour appears hypointense both in T1 (Fig. 11) and in T2.

Lymphoma. The localization of lymphoma can initially be extradural, with or without osseous involvement. The CT, whose aspect is relatively unspecific, shows the lesion as a mixed hypo- or hyperdense mass, in relation to the various degrees of calcification of the lesion. For the diagnosis, 4 parameters should be considered (Lyons et al. 1992): advanced age in a patient with worsening myelopathy; anamnestic negativity

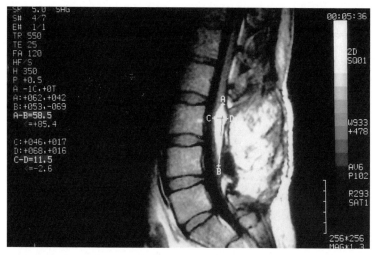

Fig. 12a. MRI T1-weighted image; sagittal view: hyperintense lesion at the level of the conus medullaris. Histology: lipoma.

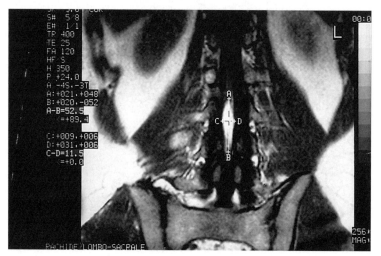

Fig. 12b. MRI T1-weighted image; coronal view: hyperintense lesion at the level of the conus medullaris. Histology: lipoma.

for other tumours; normal X-ray; extradural medullary compression with MRI that reveals a sleeve-shaped lesion (hypointense in T1-weighted images and dishomogeneously hyperintense in T2) which may involve spinal metameres.

Lipoma-Angiolipoma. These are more or less mature fat-cell tumours. The lipoma is composed of a fibrous-fat mass within the spinal canal, often associated with congenital abnormalities such as spina bifida, meningocele, myelomeningocele, dermal sinus, tethered-cord, etc. The CT shows a hypodense mass, while the MRI appearance is characterized by a relatively high signal on T1-weighted image (Figs. 12a-12b-13) and by relatively diminished signal intensity in T2-weighted image.

The angiolipoma is a tumour formed by mature fat-cells and characterized by a rich, pathological, sometimes atypical vascularization.

Hyperplastic smooth muscle cells can be present, together with osteoid or chondroid tissues. Although mostly extradural, very few cases of intramedullary angiolipoma have been reported. The CT shows a hypodense lesion with variable contrast-enhancement. The hypodensity varies in relation to the vascularization or to the presence of calcification (Preul 1993).

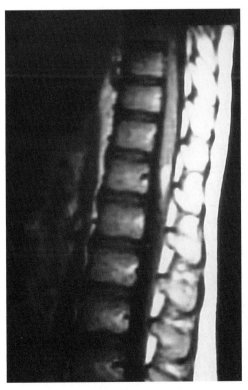

Fig. 13. MRI T1-weighted images; sagittal view: hyperintense elongated tumour at the level of the conus medullaris. Histology: lipoma.

The MRI shows a dishomogeneously iso-hyperintense mass in T1-weighted image and hyperintense in T2, in relation to the pathologic vascularization (Preul et al. 1993; Osborn 1994). Gadolinium enhancement is described in one case of intramedullary angiolipoma (Preul et al. 1993).

Intramedullary tumours

The scarce anatomical resolution of the CT does not permit easy discrimination of the morpho-structural modifications of the cord, except with the use of a subarachnoid contrast medium.

The CT thus plays a minimal role in the precocious phase of intramedullary gliomas in particular, but also in its subsequent clinico-radiological development, since even with i.v. contrast-enhancement it is difficult to distinguish the tumour from the cord parenchyma in axial cutting.

The tumour appears isodense in respect to the parenchyma without i.v. contrast-enhancement. The myelo-CT provides a greater diagnostic capability, clearly evidencing the radiological signs of subarachnoid obliteration effected by the tumour, which can be clearly imaged with this method. The CT diagnostic role is greater in cases in which these tumours have a cystic component, hypodense in relation to the parenchyma, or in non glial tumours (lipomas, teratomas, hemangioblastomas) in which the different anatomical characteristics of the tumour can have varying radiological density, visible by CT.

The CT's limits in diagnosing intramedullary gliomas also consist of the impossibility of obtaining the coronal and sagittal images that are important from a diagnostic and therapeutic point of view.

All the CT's limits in diagnosing intramedullary tumours are overcome by MRI. The spatial resolution of spinal anatomical structures and their relations are clearly evidenced even in the precocious phase, and small morpho-structural modifications are also easily evidenced by i.v. gadolinium enhancement. Moreover the possibility of obtaining images of coronal and sagittal cuts allows a suitable representation of the longitudinal extension of the lesion, and the localization in the mass of cystic intra- or peri-tumoral components.

Ependymoma. The intramedullary ependymoma appears isointense (Parizel et al. 1989) or hypointense (Schweitzer et al. 1992) in T1-weighted images (Figs. 14-15), with a marked (Fig. 16) and, at times, dishomogeneous contrast-enhancement (McCormic et al. 1990) and hyperintense in T2 (Schweitzer et al. 1992), with at times irregular hypointensity at the edges of the lesion (Fig.17) (Nemoto et al. 1992).

There may also be signs of intra- or peri-tumoral haemorrhage (Bruni et al. 1991; Chamberlain et al. 1991; Osborn 1994).

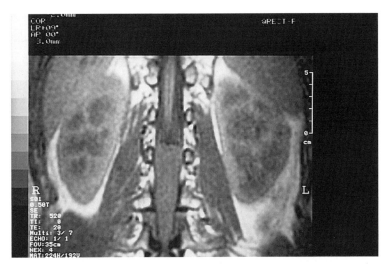

Fig. 14. MRI T1-weighted image; coronal view: isointense tumour at the level of the cauda equina. Histology: filum terminale ependymoma.

Frequently, CSF caudally to the mass appears hyperintense in T1 because of the increased proteic content (Schweitzer et al. 1992).

Astrocytoma. This has the same MRI characteristics as the ependymoma (hypo-isointense lesion in T1-weighted images with gadolinium enhancement and hyperintense in T2 (Parizel et al. 1989; Sze et al. 1990), although it may appear less demarcated (Figs. 18-19-20) (Osborn 1994).

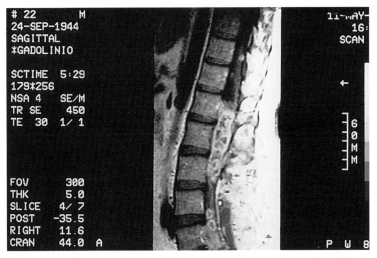

Fig. 15. MRI T1-weighted image; sagittal view: longated and multiloculated low-thoracic intramedullary tumour, with irregular hyper-hypointense pattern. Histology: ependymoma.

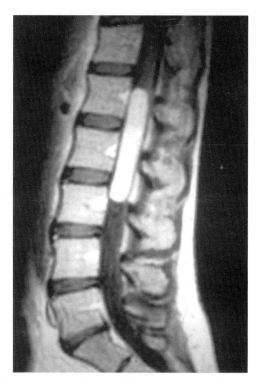

Fig. 16. MRI gadolinium enhanced T1- weighted image; sagittal view: fusiform hyperintense tumour at the level of the filum terminale. Histology: ependymoma.

Glioblastoma multiforme. The MRI aspect is difficult to differentiate from that of gliomas, described above, even if dishomogeneity in all sequences is more frequent (Ciappetta et al. 1991).

In intramedullary gliomas in which a cystic component is present, it appears hypointense in T1-weighted images and hyperintense in T2 (McCormic 1990). In T1 images the hypointensity of the cystic component is less than that of the CFS, in relation to the increased proteic content of the cystic fluid or to bleeding, and can only with difficulty be differentiated from the solid parts or from the parenchyma without a contrast medium (Brumberg et al. 1991; Chamberlain et al. 1991). In such cases a contrast-enhanced exam is indispensable, whereby it is possible to establish the real origin of the cyst (Slasky et al. 1987; Valk et al. 1988; Dillon et al. 1989). The cystic components associated with an intramedullary tumour, in relation to enhancement modalities, are divided into 3 groups (Chamberlain et al. 1991): intra-tumoral cysts (hypointense areas inside the contrast-enhanced lesion); enhanced extra-tumoral cysts (hypointense areas with a wall nodule that enhances with a contrast medium); non-enhanced extra-tumoral cysts (hypointense areas without enhancement).

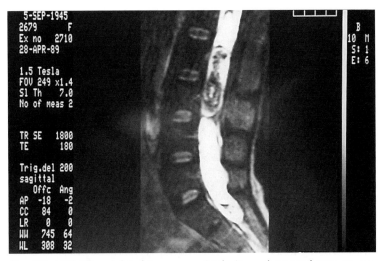

Fig. 17. MRI T2-weighted image; sagittal view: elongated tumour occupying almost the entire lumbar vertebral canal, with a central unhomogeneously isointense area and a small superior and a large inferior hyperintense portion. Histology: cono-caudal ependymoma.

Today the possibility of a differential diagnosis among intramedullary gliomas with MRI is still slight and much research has been carried out on this issue.

In differential diagnosis of the kind, i.v. contrast-enhancement modalities of the tumour have proved useful. Ependymomas are inclined to show an intense, homogeneous and clear-cut enhancement occupying the whole involved medullary seg-

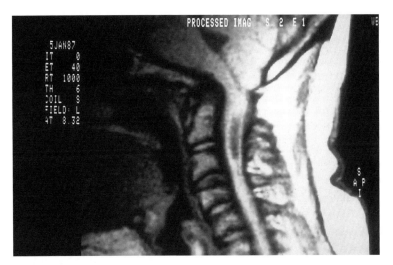

Fig. 18. MRI T1-weighted image; sagittal view: intramedullary spinal cord hypointense space-occupying mass, with fusiform shape, at C1-C3 level. Histology: astrocytoma (I WHO).

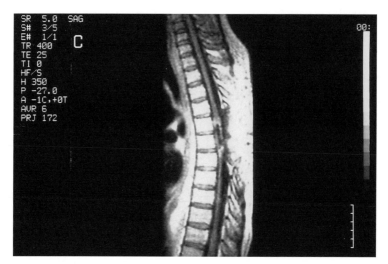

Fig. 19. MRI T1-weighted image; sagittal view: intramedullary spinal cord tumour at T6-T8 level, with a hypointense elongated central area and superior and inferior hyperintense extremities. Histology: astrocytoma (II WHO).

ment, while the astrocytomas tend to show a more irregular, spotted enhancement with irregular margins and without involving the whole medullary segment. These last aspects are to be connected with the infiltrative nature of the lesions (Parizel et al. 1989). However, ependymomas have a homogeneous enhancement pattern in only 50% of cases (above all when the images are taken 20 minutes after the injection of the contrast medium), while the remaining 50% has a dishomogeneous enhancement as in all cases of astrocytomas (Valk et al. 1988; Chamberlain et al. 1991). In conclusion, the enhancement pattern of astrocytomas and ependymomas makes differential diagnosis generally possible, even if at present the difference between the two tumours in any specific case is not totally verifiable. There seem, however, to be different enhancement patterns in the two kinds: homogeneous, clearly demarcated, and tending to occupy the whole medullary surface in the ependymoma, and dishomogeneous, irregular of margin, and eccentric with regard to the medulla in astrocytomas (Dillon et al. 1989). One case was described in which the enhancement pattern was typical of an ependymoma but the tumour was histologically an astrocytoma; another which showed the opposite (Parizel et al. 1989).

In 26 cases of histologically-diagnosed cervical intramedullary gliomas (Nemoto et al. 1992), 64% of ependymomas presented a peri-tumoral hypointense area not present in astrocytomas. This area corresponded histologically to previous bleeding. The author explains these aspects through the more frequent traction and tortion movements of the nervous cervical structures. These movements would provoke some bleeding at the surface of the tumour, absent in the astrocytoma in re-

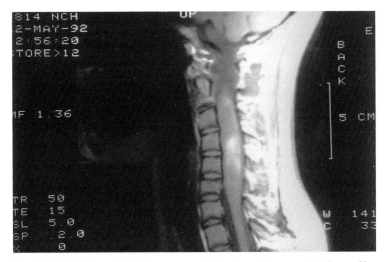

Fig. 20. MRI T1-weighted image; sagittal view: abnormal fusiform dilatation of the spinal cord at C2-C6 level, containing an irregular iso-hyperintense mass. Histology: astrocytoma (II WHO).

lation to its infiltrative nature. He concludes that hypointense peri-tumoral areas of a cervical intramedullary glioma may indicate an ependymoma.

In spite of these studies, the possibility of MRI differential diagnosis among intramedullary gliomas is still scarce, and further studies will be useful to define this important issue.

Hemangioblastoma. This is composed of a vascularized mass with hypertrophic leptomeningeal vessels; in 50-70% of cases there is a neoplastic cyst with a wall nodule. In 75% of cases it is completely intramedullary, while in other cases it may be esophitic (Osborn 1994). With MRI the tumour appears as a dishomogeneous iso-hypointense mass in T1-weighted images, and hyperintense in T2 (Silbergeld et al. 1989; Murota et al. 1989). In the images taken soon after the injection of gadolinium a clear-cut enhancement is present. Perilesional edema and, in 50% of cases, serpiginous flow-void areas are also present (Silbergeld et al. 1989; Osborn 1994).

Surgical therapy notes

Surgical results are better when the operation is performed at an early stage of the disease. The approach, the surgical technique, the radicality of removal and the consequent prognosis naturally depend not only on tumour site and histology but also on early diagnosis which, as already said, can allow the restitutio ad integrum. It is valuable for benign intradural extramedullary and intramedullary tumours (ependymomas, hemangioblastomas, etc.), while in some intramedullary neuro-epithelial tumours their infiltrative nature frequently permits only a biopsy of the lesion, with a negative prognosis quoad functionem and often quoad vitam.

Each operation is naturally preceded by careful surgical planning and the most suitable approach to the lesion has to be the result of an accurate clinical examination and evaluation of neuroimages (TC and/or MRI).

The patient's position changes in relation to the tumour site and thus to the approach planned. More often the patient is laid in prone position, in the posterior and posterolateral approaches: the surgical field must be above the heart, and the abdomen and thorax must not be compressed to avoid venous engorgement and to achieve adequate pulmonary ventilation. In the anterior approach the patient is laid in a supine or lateral position; when the tumour involves the dorsal or lumbar segments, it is particularly useful during this approach to operate with a thoracic or general surgeon. In selected cases of lesions at C1 and C2, the transoral or submandibular approach may be used.

Vertebral extradural tumours

Apart from rare benign vertebral tumours such as angiomas, osteoid osteomas, osteoblastomas, giant-cell tumours and fibroblastomas, most are malignant (metastases from carcinomas or, rarely, vertebral osteosarcoma). When the vertebral metastasis does not provoke a clinically important myelo-radicular compression and is radiosensitive, conservative management can be assumed, placing an external brace (such as a halo-vest) and prescribing for the patient oncological radio- and chemotherapy. When clinical features render it necessary (sometimes with urgency), we must operate to decompress the spinal cord and roots. Generally surgical indications for extradural metastatic tumours are as follows:

1) spinal deformity and instability which cause myelo-radicular compressions;
2) impending deformity and/or probable spinal instability;
3) intractable pain;
4) worsening of neurological deficiency during conservative management;
5) non-radiosensitive tumour (Flatley et al. 1984; Fidler 1986; Cantu 1988; Brihaye 1988).

For extradural tumours a posterior, posterolateral, anterior, anterolateral or combined approach may be used (Cantu 1988; Brihaye 1988) and is linked to the site and extension of the lesion, to the amount of metameres involved, to the patient's neurological and general conditions, to the possible vertebral instability and, of course, to the neurosurgeon's experience (Black 1985).

Often the surgical procedure, independently of the approach, is so aggressive as to provoke an instability of the involved vertebral tract, and a fusion of vertebral bodies with acrylic and/or metallic materials during the same operation is therefore indispensable (Harrington 1984; Cantu 1988; Roy-Camille et al. 1992).

In the past, myelo-radicular decompression was almost always effected by a wide laminectomy extended beyond the affected metameres, taking care to save almost the one anterior third of the facet-joint, or in any case the facet-joint on one side in order to avoid destabilizing the column (Hall and Mackai 1973). A wide review of vertebral metastases treated with posterior decompression has shown a satisfactory clinical evolution (arrest or slight improvement of neurological progression) in about 40% of cases and a definite improvement of preoperative neurological deficiency in 1/3 of cases (Black 1985). In the remaining cases, generally patients affected by anteriorly-located metastases, the laminectomy has not determined a successful decompression and has caused column district destabilization, with a consequent painful and neurologic symptomatology. Hall and Mackay (1973) observe that the laminectomy determines a clinic improvement in 39% of cases with posterior lesion, in 35% with lateral same, in 25% with a circumferential tumour and in 9% of cases with a tumour localized exclusively in the anterior epidural space.

The modern procedure is to effect laminectomy only when myelo-radicular compression is limited to the posterior vertebral arch. When the tumour is mainly localized at the pedicles and/or the facet-joint and/or vertebral bodies (the "three columns of Dennis") involving one or more contiguous metameres, with possible vertebral dislocations, the posterolateral (lateral extracavitary costotransversecto-my or lateral parascapular extracavitary costotransversoarthropedunculectomy) or transthoracic approaches are preferable. In high cervical tumours (C1-C2) transo-ral or transmandibular approaches with glossotomy or submandibular Stevenson's approaches are preferable, while at inferior cervical levels Cloward's anterolateral approach is indicated. At D1-D3 levels transternal or posterolateral parascapular extracavitary approaches are used, while at D4-D12 levels transthoracic or lateral extracavitary approaches are suggested. At D12-L1 levels we proceed through a thoraco-abdominal approach involving the section of the last three ribs and the de-tachment of the diaphragm. Lastly, anterior aggression of the lumbosacral column is effected through a retroperitoneal or intraperitoneal transabdominal approach. The level of the lesion is easily identifiable during surgery because the anterior longitudinal ligament, albeit usually intact, is segmentally raised by the tumour be-low. With a sharp dissector the anterior longitudinal ligament is removed to expose the affected vertebrae. Using a vertebral retractor, the normal intervertebral space is re-established, reducing the associated kyphosis, and the discal material re-moved. The anterior cortical of intact bodies above and below the involved level must also be exposed, to insert screws on which to secure metal bars. The neo-plastic mass is thus removed, extracting the whole of the "carious" vertebral bo-dies and exposing the anterior part of the dura mater protected by posterior longi-tudinal ligament. The sheath of roots is posterolaterally uncovered with blunt dis-section and decompressed with curettes. In doing this manoeuvre in the cervical tract, care must be taken to avoid the vertebral artery in the transversary canal. The articular plates of intact vertebral bodies have to be grooved with a high-speed drill to allow the fusion of methylmethacrylate, and to reduce the danger of polymerized acrylic material shift. The acrylic resin is inserted to fill the whole surgical field; polymerization and solidification then have to take place, taking care to avoid compressing the dura mater (Scoville et al. 1967; Dunn 1977; Harrington 1984). Anterior and anterolateral extradural tumours should therefore be treated and stabilized in the same operation through an anterior approach; the tumours involving the pedicles, laminae and spinous processes should be treated and held stabilized (if necessary) through a posterior approach; broad tumours involving both the anterior structures and the posterior ones should be removed and held stabilized (if necessary) in a single sur-gical procedure with a combined anterior and posterior approach (Cantu 1988). A pos-terior fixation with Roy-Camille's plates (in the cervical tract), with Harrington's bars (for thoracolumbar tract) or with a Diapason device (for lumbar tract) is advisable when:

a) anterior and posterior decompression is necessary;
b) the length of anterior fixation is unsuitable for restoring the correct firmness;
c) the instability is caused by surgical or neoplastic lysis of the posterior struc-tures;
d) the lesions are caudal to L3.

Anterior stabilization, with the use of acrylic material and/or osseous cement, is indicated in aggressive surgical therapies with an anterior approach, above all at cervical level, and allows a precocious mobilization of a generally elderly patient. On account of frequent radiotherapy, autologous bone wedges are rarely used in these patients (Harrington 1984).

Intradural extramedullary tumours

The surgical removal of intradural extramedullary tumours is generally effected with a posterior or posterolateral approach (Guidetti 1974; Rengachary 1993); anterior aggression is rarely necessary, although occasionally at the cranio-cervical junction and in the upper cervical tract (transoral and submandibular approaches). Intradural extramedullary tumours are generally benign (neurinomas, meningiomas); the surgeon's goal must thus be the complete removal of the tumour, presenting no difficulty at the precocious stage. Before starting the operation it is indispensable to determine the laminae corresponding to the lesion, with a radiographic label. The patient is put in the prone position, avoiding thoracoabdominal compression and consequent venous engorgement. The surgical procedure is well-known: cutting of the muscular fascia as far as the spinous processes; paravertebral muscles are then bilaterally detached and the laminae and facet-joints exposed.

The spinous processes and the laminae must be carefully removed by rongeurs or a high-speed drill. In the anterolateral tumours the removal of a part or the whole facet-joint of one side is often necessary (Rengachary 1993). It is useful also to remove the laminae above and below the lesion to allow a wider dural opening and a better control of the tumour. In hour-glass intra-extraforaminal tumours it is necessary to open the neural foramen with a high-speed drill, sacrificing part of the apophyseal mass; in these cases the intradural portion of the tumour should be removed before the extraforaminal same, to reduce manipulation and traction against the spinal cord (Rengachary 1992). Wide laminectomies, above all in childhood, can provoke later kyphosis and scoliosis; some neurological surgeons thus prefer the laminotomy to the laminectomy, repositioning the removed laminae at the end of the operation (Raimondi et al. 1976). The laminotomy, however, does not seem to reduce the secondary spinal deformity. The dura mater is opened in the midline by using an operating microscope, taking care to try to save the arachnoid plane. Then, with a microdissector, the dura is separated from the arachnoid below (Fig. 21). Generally, above all when posterior, and even at a precocious stage, the tumour is at once exposed under the arachnoid plane. The arachnoid is carefully opened with a sharp dissector and the edges coagulated or suspended. If the tumour involves a root (Fig. 22), a very accurate dissection should be made to avoid the lesion of a radiculo-medullary artery, the interruction of which can provoke ischemia of the anterior 2/3 of the spinal cord at the corresponding level, with serious clinical consequences.

It is very important not to tear the spinal cord; this is easier if the diagnosis is precocious and the tumour is small. If the diagnosis is tardy and the tumour bigger, it is preferable to alternate the dissection with a progressive reduction of the mass, using bipolar and CUSA or LASER. Debulking the lesion, the edges of the mass

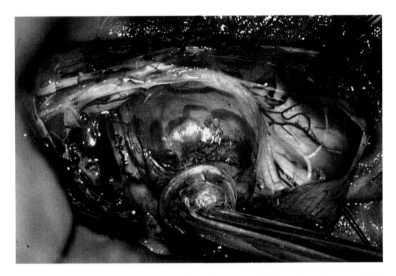

Fig. 21. Surgical aspect of an intradural extramedullary dorsal tumour. Histology: meningioma.

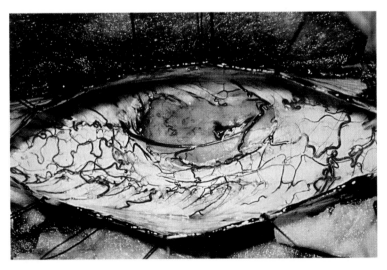

Fig. 22. Surgical aspect of an intradural extramedullary dorsal tumour. Histology: neurinoma.

shrink, making the circumferential dissection of the tumour capsule easier. When the tumour appears from a Schwann's sheath of a spinal nerve, it is sometimes necessary to cut the root or the same nerve to achieve complete removal. In the antero-lateral intradural extramedullary tumours the exposure and removal of the tumour can be made easier not only by hemiarthrectomy and costotransversectomy (Guidetti 1974; Rengachary 1993) but also by cutting the dentate ligaments and by posterior selective rizotomy (Stein 1987; Bucci and Hoff 1991).

Dural inserction of the tumour, if present, must be removed and replaced with dural plastic or, when this is impossible, must be widely coagulated with bipolar.

It is useful to remember that, before the suture of the dura, it is important to ensure an accurate haemostasis of the surgical field, and that the same suture is water-proof to avoid postoperative CSF fistula.

Intramedullary tumours

The aggression to the tumour is effected through a posterior approach (Guidetti, Fortuna et al. 1964; Stein 1987; Rengachary 1993) and the phases from the positioning of patient to the opening of the dura are the same as those described above. During surgery it is useful to record the sensory and motor-evoked potentials (Post and Stein 1988; Epstein 1993), even if the role of this recording in monitoring the medullary function is not unanimously accepted because of false positivities (Stein 1987; Brotchi et al. 1991). The whole extension of the tumour must be exposed,

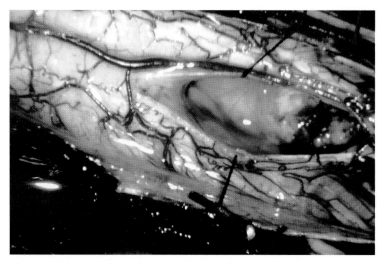

Fig. 23. Intramedullary thoracic tumour: intraoperative view after the posterior splitting of the spinal cord. Histology: ependymoma.

with the inclusion of probable cystic components. When the dura has been carefully opened, starting from the caudal pole, the spinal cord appears widened and generally with engorged veins in the caudal pole. If the tumour is evident at the dorsal or posterolateral aspect of the spinal cord, the myelotomy can be effected where the lesion is more superficial or where the cord is more enlarged (Post and Stein 1988). Intraoperative ultrasonic images can be used to localize the exact extension of the lesion (Epstein 1991; Kawakami 1992). In most cases a posterior median logitudinal myelotomy is preferable, effected with microsurgical techniques, cutting the cord with a small knife (Fig. 23). Small arterious and venous channels have to be coagulated with low intensity bipolar and under irrigation.

This procedure can be made using CO_2 LASER with focalized beam and low intensity. The myelotomy must involve the whole extension of the tumour, and the possible cleavage plane between tumour and parenchyma located and exposed. It is generally absent in astrocytomas and malignant gliomas, but almost always present in ependymomas and hemangioblastomas (Guidetti and Fortuna 1967; Stein 1987; Post and Stein 1988). There is also frequently a caudal or cranial cyst which must be emptied using a small syringe to facilitate the dissection and removal of the lesion.

In tumours with a clear cleavage plane, their edges are isolated using microsurgical technique and bipolar coagulation, or by LASER (Powers 1981). The surgical field must be kept dry in order not to lose the cleavage plane and not to damage the healthy parenchyma. In cono-caudal ependymomas it is better to remove the exophytic part of the tumour first (Stein 1987; Post and Stein 1988).

In tumours with no cleavage plane, debulking is carried out with CUSA, LASER and bipolar coagulation. Sometimes the lack of cleavage plane allows only an enlarged biopsy of the lesion (Stein 1987; Post and Stein 1988). As our and Epstein's (1992) experiences testify, total removal with microsurgical technique is possible more often than is generally thought, although the surgeon's experience is essential.

In hemangioblastomas the surgeon should not be discouraged by possible pial vessels covering the tumour, since these are easily coagulated with bipolar. The surgeon must also avoid entering the mass, which can otherwise cause severe bleeding (Guidetti and Fortuna 1964; Post and Stein 1988; Resche 1993). It is indispensable to work around the tumour, first coagulating the afferent vessels and then the main efferent veins. These tumours are often accompanied by a cyst, which facilitates their removal.

If the patient has already undergone radiotherapy a peri-tumoral gliosis is present, more evident at the rostral and caudal pole (Post and Stein 1988). This peri-tumoral gliosis makes the removal more difficult.

Conclusions

The evolution of medullary compression by spinal tumour (excepting cavernomas, vascular malformations and intramedullary hemangioblastoma) progresses, we know, in time and space, each disturbance increasing gradually, while the spinal cord is notably resistant to the slow compression.

For an early diagnosis, the analysis of the first symptom (a vertebral, radicular or cornual pain in 60% of cases) often fails to permit the correct diagnosis, since pain and paresthesias can be attributed to many osteo-articular diseases or to degenerative neurologic pathologies. The second symptom usually has a greater diagnostic value and contributes to determine an organic neurological syndrome with the characteristics of a radicular, medullary or radiculo-medullary lesion.

It should be emphasized that the average interval between the first and second symptom is about 1/4 of the average length of the disease, which means that in a short time the tumour has manifested itself through at least two symptoms, the latter of which has a greater clinical significance.

The second most frequent symptom is weakness and motor deficiency such as difficulty in walking, followed by paresthesia or hypoesthesia; in 90% of cases the precocious syndrome is thus formed by two or more symptoms causing the following associations:

- pain-paresis;
- pain-sensory disturbances;
- pain-paresis-sensory disturbances;
- paresis-sensory disturbances.

Pain is associated with other symptoms in more than 70% of cases.

In 30-40% of cases, the X-ray shows indirect signs due to bone erosion provoked by the tumour. These signs are usually absent in the precocious phase, but are, in any case, not sufficient because the neurosurgeon must preventively be sure of the tumour site, its extension and, if possible, its nature.

Today highly-diagnostic, non-invasive neuroradiologic procedures, such as CT or MRI, make such medical knowledge possible.

The precocious diagnosis of a spinal tumour is certainly possible, and can be made by the neurologist or the neurosurgeon using the above procedures; this both makes the operation easier, especially in intramedullary tumours, particularly ependymomas, and can provide the restitutio ad integrum.

Synoptic tables

FORAMEN MAGNUM TUMOURS		
SUBDURAL (extramedullary)	1) Early	- C2 radicular pain (above all neurinomas). - Disesthesias (numbness, "pins and needles" sensations, burning) in the fingers. Astereognosis in the hands. - Tetrahyperreflexia (more serious in the upper limbs).
	2) Delayed	- Hypoesthesia in the hands. - Hands-muscles atrophy (with disto-proximal evolution). - Spastic tetraparesis, more serious in the upper limbs (at times flession spasms in the lower limbs). - Superficial sensory impairment, irregularly distributed (with possible syringomyelic dissociation). - Deep hypoesthesia (more serious in the upper limbs). - C2-hypoesthesia. - Low cranial nerves deficits. - Sphincteric disturbances. - Increase of intracranial pressure.

CERVICAL TUMOURS		
SUBDURAL A) Neurinoma	1) Early	- Unilateral, monoradicular pain, sharp, persistent, often nocturnal. - Initial radicular deficit.
	2) Delayed	- Muscle radicular atrophy. - Brown-Séquard's syndrome. - Spastic paraparesis. - Sensory cordonal impairment, caudally more serious. - Sphincteric disturbances.
B) Meningioma	1) Early	- Vertebral and pluriradicular sharp pains. - Radicular paresthesias. - Initial spastic-flaccid weakness in the upper limbs. - Osteolytic lesions at X-ray. - Increase of ESR.
	2) Delayed	- Serious tetraparesis, spastic-flaccid in the upper limbs. - Cordonal hypo-anesthesia caudally more serious. - Sphincteric disturbances (rare).
INTRAMEDULLARY	1) Early	- Cornual pain; rarely monoradicular, mono/bilateral pain. - Mono/bilateral paresthesias and atrophies in upper limbs with fasciculations. - Cordonal descending pains. - Suspended hypoesthesia. - Hyperreflexia in the lower limbs.
	2) Delayed	- Serious paresis and atrophies in the upper limbs. - Spastic paraparesis. - Cordonal hypo-anesthesia, proximally more serious, with descending progression. - Sphincteric disturbances.

DORSAL TUMOURS		
SUBDURAL A) Neurinoma	1) Early	- Monoradicular pain (often misunderstood as visceral pain). - Radicular hypoesthesia. - Initial spastic paraparesis, sometimes associated with cordonal sensory deficiencies.
	2) Delayed	- Brown-Séquard's syndrome. - Spastic paraparesis. - Cordonal bilateral hypo-anesthesia, distally more serious. - Sphincteric disturbances.
B) Meningioma	1) Early	- Vertebral and radicular pains. - Cordonal paresthesias; initially distal in lower limb. - Slight mono-paraparesis. - Distal, mono-bilateral hypoesthesia.
	2) Delayed	- Brown-Séquard's syndrome. - Severe spastic paraparesis. - Cordonal bilateral hypo-anesthesia. - Sphincteric disturbances.
EXTRADURAL Malignant tumours	1) Early	- Vertebral and/or pluriradicular mono or bilateral "belt-like" pains, often misunderstood as visceral pains. - Osteolitic lesion at X-ray. - ESR increase.
	2) Delayed	- Rapidly evolving paraparesis. - Cordonal bilateral hypo-anesthesia, distally more serious. - Sphincteric disturbances.
INTRAMEDULLARY	1) Early	- Descending cordonal and vertebral pain in the thorax and/or abdomen; rare radicular or cornual pain. - Metameric hypo-anesthesia. - Spastic monoparesis.
	2) Delayed	- Spastic mono-paraparesis. - Metameric hypo-anesthesia. - Sphincteric disturbances.

CONO-FILUM TUMOURS		
SUBDURAL A) Neurinoma	1) Early	- Radicular sciatic pain with negativity of Lasègue's sign. - Mono or bilateral paresis and atrophies in lower limbs with fasciculations. - Radicular or cordonal hypoesthesia.
	2) Delayed	- Flaccid or spastic paraparesis. - Radicular and/or cordonal sensory deficiency, more serious at the perineum. - Sphincteric disturbances.
B) Meningioma	1) Early	- Slight pluriradicular mono or bilateral pains. - Radicular or cordonal paresthesias. - Slight flaccid or spastic paraparesis. - Slight pluriradicular and/or metameric sensory deficiencies.
	2) Delayed	- Flaccid or spastic paraparesis. - Hypo-anesthesia more serious at the perineum. - Sphincteric disturbances.
EXTRADURAL Malignant tumours	1) Early	- Sharp vertebral and pluriradicular pains. - Flaccid and spastic paresis. - Pluriradicular or cordonal sensory deficiency. - ESR increase.
	2) Delayed	- Serious flaccid paraparesis. - Serious hypo-anesthesia. - Sphincteric disturbances.
INTRAMEDULLARY	1) Early	- Pseudosciatalgia (undefined, nocturnal, burning pain with negativity of Lasègue's sign). - Fasciculations in the lower limbs. - Irregularly-distributed spastic-flaccid motor deficiencies in the lower limbs.
	2) Delayed	- Flaccid-spastic paraparesis with atrophies in the lower limbs. - Irregularly-distributed hypo-anesthesia. - Sphincteric disturbances.

REFERENCES

ABBOTT K.H.: *Subarachnoid haemorrage from an ependymoma arising in the filum terminale. Report of a case.* Bull Los Angeles Neurol. Soc. 4: 127-132, 1939.

ADSON A.W.: *Tumours of the spinal cord. Diagnosis and treatment.* Canad. Med. Ass. 40: 448-461, 1939.

AFSHAR F.: *Syringomyelia and spinal cord tumours.* Curr. Opin. Neurology Neurosurg. 3: 581-584, 1990.

AHYAI A., WOERNER U., MARKAKIS E.: *Surgical treatment of intramedullary tumors (spinal cord and medulla oblongata). Analysis of 16 cases.* Neurosurg. Rev. 13: 45-52, 1990.

ALBRECHT S., CRUTCHFIELD J., SEGALL G.: *On spinal osteochondromas.* J. Neurosurg. 77: 247-252, 1992.

ALEMÀ G.: *Il tipo pseudomiotonico di apertura della mano nelle ernie del disco cervicale.* Riv. di Neurol. 28: 631-634, 1958.

ALLEN J., LASSOFF S.: *Outcome after surgery for intramedullary spinal cord tumours.* Neurosurgery 26: 1091, 1990 (Letter).

ALP H., CEVIKER N., BAYKANER K. ET AL.: *Osteoblastoma of the third lumbar vertebra.* Surg. Neurol. 9: 276-279, 1983.

ALTER M.: *Statistical aspects of spinal cord tumours.* In: VINKEN P.J., BRUYN G.W., *Handbook of Clinical Neurology*, vol. 19, part 1: "Tumours of the spine and spinal cord", pp. 1-22, North-Holland Publishing Company, Amsterdam, North-Holland, 1975.

ALVISI C., CERISOLI M., GIULIONI M.: *Intramedullary spinal gliomas: Long-term results of surgical Treatments.* Acta Neurochir. 70: 169-179, 1984.

AL WAHHABI B., CHOUDHURY A., CHAUDHRI K. ET AL: *Multicentric glioma of the spinal cord.* Br. J. Neurosurg. 6: 495-499, 1992.

AMACHER A.L., ELTOMEY A.: *Spinal osteoblastoma in children and adolescents.* Child's Nerv. Syst. 1: 29-32, 1985.

AMICI R., BORGHI G.P.: *Emorragia subarcnoidea da tumori spinali intradurali del tratto lombare.* Min. Neurochirurgica 3: 191-198, 1959.

ANDERSEN S., SAMUELSSON L.: *Spinal metastases - Survival and neurological improvement after laminectomy.* Acta Orthop. Scand. 62: 19-20, 1991.

ANDRÉ-THOMAS T., FERRAND J., SCHAFFER H., DE MARTEL D.: *Syndrome d'emorragie meningee realisé par un tumeur de la quene de cheval.* Presse Mèd. 77: 292-298, 1930.

ANSON J., CYBULSKI G., REYES M.: *Spinal extradural angiolipoma: a report of two cases and review of the literature.* Surg. Neurol. 34: 173-178, 1990.

ANTONI N.R.E.: *Ueber Ruckenmarkstumoren und Neurofibroma.* München ed., 1920.

AOKI J., MORIYA K., YAMASHITA K. ET AL.: *Giant cell tumours of bone containing large amounts of haemosiderin: MR-Pathologic correlation.* J. Compt. Asst. Tomogr. 15: 1024-1027, 1991.

ARGUELLO F., BAGGS R., DUERST R. ET AL.: *Pathogenesis of vertebral metastasis and epidural spinal cord compression.* Cancer 65: 98-106, 1990.

ARSENI C., DANAILA L., COSTANTINESCU A., CARP N.: *Spinal dermoid tumours.* Neurochirurgia (Stuttg.) 20: 108-116, 1977.

ARSENI C., IONESCO S.: *Les compressions médullaires dues à des tumeurs intrarachidiennes Etude clinico-statistique de 362 cases.* J. Chir. Paris 75: 582-594, 1958.

ARSENI C., SIMONESCU M., HORWATH L.: *Tumours of the spine.* Acta Psychiat. Scand. 34: 398-410, 1959.

AUBERGE C., PONSOT G., LEMERLE J. ET AL.: *Tumeurs intramedullaires de l'enfant.* Arch. Fr. Pediatr. 36: 1024-1039, 1979.

AULISA L., TAMBURRELLI F., GALLI M.: *Osteoblastoma of the atlas.* Child's Nerv. Syst. 9: 115-116, 1993.

AUSTIN G.M.: *The significance and nature of the pain in tumours of the spinal cord.* Surg. Forum 10: 782-785, 1960.

AUSTIN G.M.: *The spinal cord.* Third Edition, Igaku-Shoin, New York, Tokio, pp. 833, 1983.

AWWAD E., BACKER R., ARCHER C.: *The imaging of an intraspinal cervical dermoid tumour by MR, CT and sonography.* Comput. Radiol. 11: 169-173, 1987.

AYSUN S., CINBIS M., OZCAN O.: *Intramedullary astrocytoma presenting as spinal muscular atrophy.* J. Child. Neurol. 8: 354-356, 1993.

AZOUZ E., KOZLOWSKI K., MARTON D. ET AL.: *Osteoid osteoma and osteoblastoma of the spine in children.* Pediatr. Radiol. 16: 25-31, 1986.

BACCI G., PICCI P., CALDERONI P.: *Full-lung tomograms and bone scanning in the initial workup of patient with osteogenic sarcoma: a review of 126 cases.* Eur. J. Cancer. 18: 967-971, 1982.

BAILEY J.: *Dermoid tumours of the spinal cord.* J. Neurosurg. 33: 676-681, 1970.

BAKER N., GREENSPAN A., NEUWIRTH M.: *Symptomatic vertebral haemangiomas: a report of four cases.* Skeletal. Radiol. 15: 458-463, 1986.

BAKER L., GOODMAN S., PERKASH I.: *Benign versus pathological compression fractures of vertebral bodies: assessment with conventional spin-echo chemical-shift and STIR MR imaging.* Radiology 174: 495-502, 1990.

BALAGURA S.: *Late neurological dysfunction in adult lumbosacral lipoma with tethered cord.* Neurosurgery 15: 724-726, 1984.

BARCENA A., LOBATO R., RIVAS J. ET AL.: *Spinal metastatic disease: analysis of factors determining functional prognosis and the choice of treatment.* Neurosurgery 15: 820-827, 1984.

BARDELLA L., ARTICO M., NUCCI F.: *Intramedullary subependymoma of the cervical spinal cord.* Surg. Neur. 29: 326-329, 1988.

BARONE B., ELVIDGE A.: *Ependymomas. A clinical survey.* J. Neurosurg. 33: 428-438, 1970.

BELTRAN J., NOTO A., CHAKERES D., CHRISTOFORIDIS A.: *Tumours of the osseous spine: staging with MR imaging versus CT.* Radiology 162: 565-569, 1987.

BENZEL E., MIRFARKHRAEE M., HADDEN T., FOWLER M.: *Holocord astrocytoma: a two-staged operative approach.* Spine 12: 746-749, 1987.

BERCIANO J., GUTIERREZ J., REBOLLO M., DIERSSEN G.: *Thoracic spinal cord ependymoma presenting with ejaculatory failure. Case report.* J. Neurosurg. 56: 143-144, 1982.

BERNAT J., GREENBERG E., BARRETT J.: *Suspected epidural compression of the spinal cord and cauda equina by metastatic carcinoma clinical diagnosis and survival.* Cancer 51: 1953-1957, 1983.

BLAK P.: *Spinal epidural tumours.* In: WILKINS R.H., RENGACHARY S.S., *Neurosurgery*, vol. 1, cap. 126, McGraw-Hill, Book Company, 1985.

BLAND L.: *Osteochondroma of the vertebral column.* Neurosurgery 27: 660-668, 1990.

BLAYLOCK R.: *Hydrosyringomyelia of the conus medullaris associated with a thoracic meningioma: case report.* J. Neurosurg. 54: 833-835, 1981.

BOCCARDO M., RUELLE A., MARIOTTI E., SEVERI P.: *Spinal carcinomatous metastases. Retrospective study of 67 surgically treated cases.* J. Neuroncol. 3: 251-257, 1985.

BOLDREY E., ELVIDGE A.: *Dermoid cysts of the vertebral canal.* Ann. Surg. 110: 273-284, 1939.

BOOGERD W., VAN DER SANDE J., KROGER R.: *Early diagnosis and treatment of spinal epidural metastasis in breast cancer: a prospective study.* J. Neurol. Neurosurg. Psychiatry 55: 1188-1193, 1992.

BORGHI G.: *Extradural spinal meningiomas.* Acta Neurochir. 29: 195-202, 1973.

BOROVICH B., KERET D., BEN-ARIE J. ET AL.: *Spinal intradural metastases of extraneural origin.* Acta Neurochir. 56: 99-105, 1981.

BOUGHEY A., FLETCHER N., HARDING A.: *Central nervous system haemangioblastoma: a clinical and genetic study of 52 cases.* J. Neurol. Neurosurg. Psychiatry 53: 644-648, 1990.

BOYD H.: *Iatrogenic intraspinal epidermoid. Report of a case.* J. Neurosurg. 24: 105-107, 1966.

BRAUNSTEIN E., KUHNS L.: *Computed tomographic demonstration of spinal metastases.* Spine 8: 912-915, 1983.

BREGER R., WILLIAMS A., DANIELS D. ET AL.: *Contrast enhancement in spinal MR imaging.* Am. J. Neuroradiol. 10: 633-637, 1989.

BREUER A., KNEISLEY L., FISCHER E.: *Treatable extramedullary cord compression. Meningioma as a cause of Brown-Séquard's syndrome.* Spine 5: 19-22, 1980.

BRIHAYE J., ECTORS P., LEMONT M., VAN HOUTTE P.: *The management of spinal epidural metastases.* Advances and Technical Standard in Neurosurgery, vol. 16: 122-176, Springer-Verlag, Wien-New York, 1988.

BROADDUS W., GRADY M., DELASHAW J. JR ET AL.: *Preoperative superselective arteriolar embolization: a new approach to enhance resectability of spinal tumours.* Neurosurgery 27: 755-759, 1990.

BROAGER B.: *Spinal neurinoma*. Acta Psychiatr. Neurol. 85: 1-241, 1953.

BROTCHI J., DEWITTE O., LEVIVIER M. ET AL.: *A survey of 65 tumours within the spinal cord: surgical results and the importance of preoperative magnetic resonance imaging.* Neurosurgery 29: 651-657, 1991.

BROWNE T., ADAMS R., ROBERSON G.H.: *Haemangioblastoma of spinal cord.* Arch. Neurol. 33: 435-441, 1976.

BRUNBERG J., DI PIETRO M., VENES J. ET AL.: *Intramedullary lesions of the pediatric spinal cord: correlation of findings from MR imaging, intraoperative sonography, surgery and histologic study.* Radiology 181: 573-579, 1991.

BRUNI P., ESPOSITO S., ODDI G. ET AL.: *Subarachnoid haemorrhage from multiple neurofibroma of the cauda equina: case report.* Neurosurgery 28: 910-913, 1991.

BUCCI M.N., HOFF J.T.: *Spinal meningiomas.* In: RENGACHARY S.S., WILKINS R.H. (eds), *Neurosurgical Operative Atlas*, vol. 1, pp. 123-126, Williams & Wilkins, Baltimore, 1991.

BULL J.: *Spinal meningiomas and neurofibromas.* Acta Radiol. 40: 283-300, 1991.

BUTTI G., GAETANI P., SCELSI M., PEZZOTTA S.: *Extradural spinal lipomas. Report of two cases and review of the literature.* Neurochirurgia (Stuttg.) 27: 28-30, 1984.

BYDDER G., BROWN Y., LIEONDORF H., YOUND I.: *Enhancement of intraspinal tumours in MRI with intravenous Gadolinium-Dtpa.* J. Comput. Assist. Tomogr. 9: 847-852, 1985.

BYRNE T.: *Current concepts: spinal cord compression from epidural metastases.* New Engl. J. Med. 327: 614-619, 1992.

CAMPANACCI M., CERVELLATI G.: *Osteosarcoma. A review of 345 cases.* Ital. J. Orthop. Traumatol. 1: 5-22, 1975.

CANTORE G.P., VALENTINO V., DELFINI R.: *Diagnosi e trattamento dei tumori vertebro-midollari cervicali.* In: *Patologia del Rachide Cerevicale*, Idelson, Napoli pp. 239-243, 1985.

CANTORE G.P., DELFINI R., INNOCENZI G.: *Intramedullary tumours: problems and controverses.* Critical Review in Neurosurgery 4: 358-365, 1994.

CANTU R.C.: *Osseus fusion of the cervical, thoracic and lumbar spine with primary and metastatic spine tumours.* In: SUNDARESAN (ed.), *Tumours of the spine*, sect. C, cap. 44, pp. 446-456, 1990.

CARMODY R., YANG P., SEELEY G. ET AL.: *Spinal cord compression due to metastatic disease: diagnosis with MR imaging versus myelography.* Radiology 173: 225-229, 1989.

CARO P., MARKS H., KERET D.: *Intraspinal epidermoid tumours in children: problems in recognition and imaging technique for diagnosis.* J. Ped. Orthopaed. 11: 288-293, 1991.

CARTA F., SILVESTRO C., BORZONE M. ET AL.: *Multiple spinal meningiomas. Report of 2 cases.* Zentralbl. Neurochir. 44: 3-6, 1983.

CASSINARI V., BERNASCONI V.: *Tumori e malformazioni vasali spinali.* Acta Neurochir. 9: 612-658, 1961.

CAWTHON D., CACAYORIN E., MODESTI L. ET AL.: *Spinal vascular tumours: dilemmas in diagnosis and management.* Neurosurgery 16: 625-629, 1985.

CECCHINI A., GOZZOLI L.: *Neuroradiological aspects in primitive and metastatic spinal tumours.* Minerva Med. 75: 1345-1354, 1984.

CECCONI L., POMPILI A., CAROLI F., SQUILLACI E.: *Atlante di Risonanza Magnetica dei Tumori del Sistema Nervoso.* Edizioni Luigi Pozzi, 1992.

CELLI P., CERVONI L., CANTORE G.: *Ependymoma of the filum terminale: treatment and prognostic factors in a series of 28 cases.* Acta Neurochir. 124: 99-103, 1993.

CEREJO A., VAZ R., FEYO B.P., CRUZ C.: *Spinal cord haemangioblastoma with subarachnoid haemorrhage.* Neurosurgery 27: 991-993, 1990.

CHALIF D., BLACK K., ROSENSTEIN D.: *Intradural spinal cord tumor presenting as a subarachnoid haemorrhage Magnetic Resonance Imaging diagnosis.* Neurosurgery 27: 631-634, 1990.

CHAMBERLAIN M., SANDY A., PRESS G.: *Spinal cord tumors: gadolinium-dtpa-enhanced MR imaging.* Neuroradiology 33: 469-474, 1991.

CHAPARRO M., YOUNG R., SMITH M. ET AL.: *Multiple spinal meningiomas: a case of 47 distinct lesions in the absence of neurofibromatosis or identified chromosomal abnormality.* Neurosurgery 32: 298-302, 1992.

CHENG M.: *Spinal cord tumours in the People's Republic of China: a statistical review.* Neurosurgery 10: 22-24, 1982.

CHIGASAKI H., PENNYBACKER J.B.: *A long follow-up study of 128 cases of spinal cord tumours.* Neurologia medico-chirurgica 10: 22-26, 1968. Reprinted from: The Japanese Neurosurgical Society 10, 1968.

CHODKIEWICZ J., COSTANS J., SCHWEISGUTHO: *Les compression mèdullaires par tumeurs intrararachidienne malignes extradurales de l'enfante.* Neurochirurgie 16: 41-50, 1970.

CHOREMIS C., ECONOMOS D., PAPADATOS C., GARGOULAS A.: *Intraspinal epidermoid tumours (cholesteatomas) in patients treated for tuberculous meningitis.* Lancet 2: 437-439, 1958.

CHUN H.C., SCHMIDT-ULLRICH R.K., WOLFSON A. ET AL.: *External beam radiotherapy for primary spinal cord tumours.* J. Neuro-Oncol. 9: 211-217, 1990.

CIAPPETTA P., SALVATI M., CAPOCCIA G., ARTICO M., RACO A., FORTUNA A.: *Spinal glioblastomas: report of seven cases and review of the literature.* Neurosurgery 28: 302-306, 1991.

COLLIGNON J., KALANGU K., FLANDROY P.: *Benign osteoblastoma of the spine report on 4 cases with one spontaneous cure.* Neurochirurgia 34: 262-270, 1988.

COLMAN L., PORTER B., REDMOND J. ET AL.: *Early diagnosis of spinal metastases by CT and MR studies.* J. Comput. Assisted Tomography 12: 423-426, 1988.

COMPAGNONI L., NAPPO A., SALVATORI G.: *Intraspinal metastases.* Neurology 40: 1146-1147, 1990.

CONNOLLY E.: *Spinal cord tumours in adults.* In: YOUMANS Jr (ed.), *Neurological Surgery Philadelphia.* Wb Saunders, pp. 3196-3214, 1982.

CONSTANS J., DE DIVITIIS E., DONZELLI R. ET AL.: *Spinal metastases with neurological manifestations. Review of 600 cases.* J. Neurosurg. 59: 111-118, 1983.

CONTI P., CONTI R., LO RE F.: *2 rare cases of intraspinal meningioma in childhood.* Riv. Neurobiol. 27: 536-542, 1981.

COOPER P., EPSTEIN F.: *Radical resection of intramedullary spinal cord tumours in adults. Recent experience in 29 patients.* J. Neurosurg. 63: 492-499, 1985.

COOPER P.: *Outcome after operative treatment of intramedullary spinal cord tumours in adults: intermediate and long-term results in 51 patients.* Neurosurgery 25: 855 859, 1989.

CORADDU M., NURCHI G., FLORIS F., MELEDDU V.: *Surgical treatment of extradural spinal cord compression due to metastatic tumours.* Acta Neurochir. 111: 18-21, 1991.

COSTABILE G., PROBST C.: *Intramedullary subarachnoid epidermoid cyst with secondary purulent infection.* Neurochirurgia 26: 53-55, 1983.

CRAIG W.: *Tumours of the spinal cord.* Surg. Clin. North America 15: 1371-1382, 1935.

CRISTOFORI L., CAMPELLO M., TALACCHI A., BRICOLO A.: *La diagnosi precoce dei tumori intramidollari: analisi retrospettiva di 113 casi.* Edizioni Minerva Medica Torino, pp. 267-278, 1991.

CROCKARD A.: *Surgery for anterior placed meningiomas at the foramen magnum.* In: *Meningiomas and their surgical management.* Edited by Schmidek H.H., pp. 471-479, WB Saunders Co., Philadelphia, 1991.

CULVER G., CONCANNON J., KOENIG E.: *Calcification in intraspinal meningioma.* AJR 62: 237-246, 1949.

CYBULSKI G., VON ROENN K., D'ANGELO C., DEWALD R.: *Luque rod stabilization for metastatic disease of the spine.* Surg. Neurol. 28: 277-283, 1987.

CYBULSKI G.: *Methods of surgical stabilization for metastatic disease of the spine.* Neurosurgery 25: 240-252, 1989.

CZORNY A., BERCHET T., COUDANE H. ET AL.: *Solitary osteochondroma of spine. Report of 4 cases.* Neurochirurgie 31: 303-308, 1985.

DAGI T., SCHMIDEK H.: *Vascular tumours of the spine.* In: SUNDARESAN N., SCHMIDEK H., SCHILLER A., ROSENTHAL D., *Tumours of the spine. Diagnosis and clinical management.* WB Saunders Company, pp. 181-191, 1990.

DAHILIN D., COVENTRY M.: *Osteogenic sarcoma: a study of 600 cases.* J. Bone Joint Surg. 49a: 101-110, 1967.

DANDY W.E.: *The diagnosis and localization of spinal cord tumours.* Ann. Surg. 81: 223-230, 1925.

DARAS M., KOPPEL B., HEISE C. ET AL.: *Multiple spinal intradural schwannomas in the absence of von Recklinghausen's disease.* Spine 18: 2556-2559, 1993.

DAVIDSON H., OUCHI T., STEINER R.: *NMR imaging of congenital intracranial germinal layer neoplasms.* Neuroradiology 27: 301-303, 1985.

DAVIS R., WASHBURN P.: *Spinal cord meningiomas.* Surg. Gynecol. Obstet. 131: 15-21, 1970.

DE CARO R., GIORDANO R., PARENTI A., ZUCCARELLO: *Osteomatous meningioma. Report of two cases.* Acta Neurochir. 60: 313-317, 1982.

DECKER R., SUNDRANI S., CITRON M., HERRSCHAFT D.: *Intramedullary spinal cord metastases treated by complete resection of tumor prior to radiotherapy and chemotherapy. Case report and review.* Spine 12: 393-395, 1987.

DE DIVITIIS E., CERILLO A., CARLOMAGNO S.: *Subpial spinal lipomas.* Neurochirurgia (Stuttg.) 25: 14-18, 1982.

DE DIVITIIS E., MAIURI F., CORRIERO G., DONZELLI R.: *Subarachnoid haemorrhage due to a spinal neurinoma.* Surg. Neurol. 24: 187-190, 1985.

DE SANTOS L., BERNARDINO M., MURRAY J.: *Computed tomography in the evaluation of osteosarcoma: experience with 25 cases.* AJR 132: 535-540, 1979.

DE SOUSA L., KALSBECK J., MEALEY J. ET AL.: *Intraspinal tumours in children.* J. Neurosurg. 51: 437-445, 1979.

DEVADIGA K., GASS H.: *Multiple spinal cord meningiomas.* Neurol. India 20: 142-144, 1972.

DI CHIRO G., RIETH K., OLDFIELD E. ET AL.: *Digital subtraction angiography and dynamic computed tomography in the evaluation of arteriovenous malformations and haemangioblastomas of the spinal cord.* J. Comput. Assist. Tomogr. 6: 655-670, 1982.

DI CHIRO G., DOPPMAN J., DWYER A. ET AL.: *Tumours and arteriovenous malformations of the spinal cord: assessment using MR.* Radiology 156: 689-697, 1985.

DILLON W.P., NORMAN D., NEWTON T.H. ET AL.: *Intradural spinal cord lesions: Gd-Dtpa-enhanced MR imaging.* Radiology 170: 229-237, 1989.

DI LORENZO N., FORTUNA A., GUIDETTI B.: *Craniovertebral junction malformations. Clinico-radiological analysis, long term results and surgical indications in 63 cases.* J. Neurosurg. 57: 603-608, 1982.

DI LORENZO N., GIUFFRÈ R., FORTUNA A.: *Primary spinal neoplasms in childhood: analysis of 1234 published cases (including 56 personal cases) by pathology, sex, age and site. Differences from the situation in adults.* Neurochirurgia (Stuttg.) 25: 153-164, 1982.

DI LORENZO N., NOLLETTI A., NARDI P., FORTUNA A.: *Chondromes et osteochondrome solitarie du rachis entrainant une compression myeloradiculaire. A propos de 6 cases traites chirurgicalement.* Neurochirurgie 29: 271-278, 1983.

DI LORENZO N., NARDI P., CIAPPETTA P., FORTUNA A.: *Benign tumours and tumourlike conditions of the spine. Radiological features, treatment, and results.* Surg. Neurol. 25: 449-456, 1986.

DI LORENZO N., DELFINI R., CIAPPETTA P., CANTORE G.P., FORTUNA A.: *Primary tumours of the cervical spine: surgical experience with 38 cases.* Surg. Neurol. 38: 12-18, 1992.

DINAKAR I., SUNDARAM C., RATNAKAR K., KISHORE L.: *Extramedullary glioma of the cervicodorsal spinal cord: a case report.* Surg. Neurol. 41: 235-237, 1994.

DJINDJIAN M.: *Spinal meningeal haemorrage due to tumours: a report of 5 cases with arteriography.* Revue Neurol. 34: 685-692, 1978.

DODGE H., SVIEN H., CAMP J. ET AL.: *Tumours of the spinal cord without neurological manifestation, producing low back and sciatic pain.* Proc. Staff Meet Mayo Clinic. 26: 88-95, 1951.

DODGE H., LOVE J.G., GOTTLIEB J.: *Benign tumours at the foramen magnum.* J. Neurosurg. 13: 603-617, 1956.

DONOGHUE V., CHUANG S., CHILTON S. ET AL.: *Intraspinal epidermoid cysts.* J. Comput. Assist. Tomogr. 8: 143-144, 1984.

DONOVAN POST M., QUENCER R., GREEN B. ET AL.: *Intramedullary spinal cord metastases, mainly of non-neurogenic origin.* AJN 8: 339-346, 1987.

DOOMS G., HRICAK H., SOLLITO R., HIGGINS C.: *Lipomatous tumours and tumours with fatty component: MR imaging potential and comparison of MR on CT results.* Radiology 157: 479-483, 1985.

DORWART R., LA MASTERS D., WATANABE T.: *Tumours.* In: NEWTON T.H., POTTS D.G., *Computed tomography of the spine and spinal cord.* Clavadel Press San Anselmo 1983, pp. 115-147.

DOUGLAS F., McDONALD J., McLEOD R., UNNI K.: *Giant cell tumours of the spine and sacrum.* In: SUNDARESAN N., SCHMIDEK HH., SCHILLE A., ROSENTHAL D., *Tumours of the spine. Diagnosis and clinical management.* WB Saunders Company, 1990, pp. 173-180.

Ducati A., Rychlicki F., Scarpelli M. et al.: *Tumori intramidollari: Inquadramento clinico-patologico.* Edizioni Minerva Medica, Torino, pp. 235-245, 1991.

Dunn E.J.: *The role of methylacrylate in stabilization and replacement of tumours of the cervical spine. A project of the Cervical Spine Research Society.* Spine 2: 15-24, 1977.

Dusser D., Barenne J.G.: *Strichninwerkung auf das Zentralnervensystem.* Folia Neur. Biol. 7: 549-561, 1913.

Early C., Sayers M.: *Spinal epidural meningioma. Case report.* J. Neurosurg. 25: 571-573, 1966.

Ectors L., Achslogh J., Saintes M.J.: *Les compressions de la moelle cervicale.* Paris, Masson, 1960.

Eeg Olofsson O., Carlsson E., Jeppsson S.: *Recurrent abdominal pains as the first symptom of a spinal cord tumour.* Acta Paediatr. Scand. 70: 595-597, 1981.

Eggert H.R., Scheremet R., Seeger W., Gaitzsch J.: *Unilateral microsurgical approaches to extramedullary spinal tumours. Operative technique and results.* Acta Neurochir. 67: 245-253, 1983.

Ehni G., Love J.: *Intraspinal lipomas. Report of cases, review of the literature and clinical and pathologic study.* Arch. Neurol. Psychiatry 53: 1-28, 1945.

Elsberg C., Beer E.: *The operability of intramedullary tumours of the spine.* Am. J. Med. Sci. 142: 636-647, 1911.

Elsberg C.: *Diagnosis and treatment of surgical disease of the spinal cord and its membranes.* WB Saunders Company, pp. 330, 1916.

Elsberg C.: *Tumours of the spinal cord and the symptoms of irritation and compression of the spinal cord and nerve roots. Pathology, Symptomatology, Diagnosis and Treatment.* Paul B. Hoeber, New York, pp. 421, 1925.

Elsberg C.: *Surgical disease of spinal cord, membranes and nerve root: symptoms, diagnosis and treatment.* New York, Hoeber, Vol. 1, pp. 598, 1941.

Elsenburg P., Mauser H., Veiga Pires J., Van Veelen C.: *Panmedullary ependymoma with multiple cysts complicated by fatty deposits in the proximal spinal cord.* Clin. Neurol. Neurosurg. 85: 273-279, 1983.

Emery J., Lendon R.: *Lipomas of the cauda equina and other fatty tumours related to neurospinal dysraphism.* Dev. Med. Child. Neurol. [Suppl.] 20: 62-70, 1969.

Enomoto H., Shibata T., Ito A.: *Multiple haemangioblastomas accompained by syringomyelia in the cerebellum and the spinal cord. Review and report of five cases.* Surg. Neurol. 22: 197-303, 1984.

Epstein F., Epstein N.: *Surgical management of holocord intramedullary spinal cord astrocytomas in children. Report of three cases.* J. Neurosurg. 54: 829-832, 1981.

Epstein F., Epstein N.: *Surgical treatment of spinal cord astrocytomas of childhood. A series of 19 patients.* J. Neurosurg. 57: 685-689, 1982.

Epstein F., Epstein N.: *Intramedullary tumours of the spinal cord.* In: *Section of pediatric neurosurgery of the American Association of Neurological Surgeons* (eds), Pediatric Neurosurgery Surgery of The Developing Nervous System. New York, Grune & Stratton, pp. 529-538, 1982.

Epstein F.: *The cavitron ultrasonic aspirator in tumour surgery.* Clin. Neurosurg. 31: 497-505, 1983.

Epstein F., Wisoff J.: *Surgical management of spinal cord astrocytomas in childhood.* Riv. Neurosc. Pediatr. 1: 77-83, 1985.

Epstein F.: *Spinal cord astrocytomas in children.* Advances and Technical Standard in Neurosurgery vol. 13: 135-169, 1986; Springer-Verlag, Wien-New York.

Epstein F.: *Spinal cord astrocytomas of childhood.* Prog. Exp. Tumour Res. 30: 135-153, 1987.

Epstein F., Wisoff J.: *Intra axial tumours of the cervicomedullary junction.* J. Neurosurg. 67: 483-487, 1987.

Epstein F., Lassoff S., Wisoff J. et al.: *Primary intramedullary spinal cord tumours in children: the long-term follow-up.* J. Neurosurg. 72: 358a, 1990.

Epstein F., Farmer J.: *Trends in surgery: Laser surgery, use of the Cavitron, and debulking surgery.* Neurol. Clin. 9: 307-315, 1991.

Epstein F., Farmer J., Schneider S.: *Intraoperative ultrasonography: an important surgical adjunct for intramedullary tumours.* J. Neurosurg. 74: 729-733, 1991.

EPSTEIN F., FARMER J., FREED D.: *Adult intramedullary astrocytomas of the spinal cord*. J. Neurosurg. 77: 355-359, 1992.

EPSTEIN F., FARMER J., FREED D.: *Adult intramedullary spinal cord ependymomas: the results of surgery in 38 patients*. J. Neurosurg. 79: 204-209, 1993.

EVARD M., PASSY U.: *von Recklinghausen's disease with multiple meningiomas*. Laryngoscope 82: 2222-2225, 1972.

FACCHIN P., DE NARDI F., MEO A., CECOTTO C.: *Considerazioni clinico-terapeutiche sui tumori disontogenetici del sistema nervoso centrale*. Riv. Neurobiol. 32: 35-46, 1986.

FAERBER E., WOLPERT S.: *The value of computed tomography in the diagnosis of intracranial lipomata*. J. Comput. Assist. Tomogr. 2: 297-299, 1985.

FARWELL J., DOHRMANN G.: *Intraspinal neoplasm in children*. Paraplegia 15: 262-273, 1977.

FEARNSIDE M., ADAMS C.: *Tumours of the cauda equina*. J. Neurol. Neurosurg. Psychiatry 41: 24-31, 1978.

FEIRING E., BARRON K.: *Late recurrence of spinal cord meningiomas*. J. Neurosurg. 19: 652-656, 1962.

FERRANTE L., MASTRONARDI L., ACQUI M., FORTUNA A.: *Postoperative arachnoidal diverticula of the lumbar spine*. J. Neurosurg. Sci. 32: 131-134, 1988.

FERRANTE L., MASTRONARDI L., LUNARDI P., PUZZILLI F., FORTUNA A.: *Lumbar disk herniation in teenagers*. European Spine Journal 1: 25-28, 1992.

FERRANTE L., MASTRONARDI L., ACQUI M., MISSORI P., TACCONI L., FORTUNA A.: *Cervicomedullary junction haemangioblastoma: report of a case and review of the literature*. J. Neurosurg. Sci. 36: 59-65, 1992.

FERRANTE L., MASTRONARDI L., CELLI P., LUNARDI P., ACQUI M., FORTUNA A.: *Intramedullary spinal cord ependymomas. A study of 45 cases with long-term follow-up*. Acta Neurochir. 119: 74-79, 1992.

FERREIRA N., CHAVES D., MORAES A., DE OLIVEIRA L.: *Spinal tumours: a propos of 100 cases*. Arq. Neuropsiquiatr. 39: 25-31, 1981.

FIDLER M.W.: *Anterior decompression and stabilization of metastatic spinal fractures*. J. Bone Joint Surg. 68B.: 83-89, 1986.

FIELDING J.W., PYLE R.N., FIETTI V.G. JR: *Anterior cervical vertebral body resection and bonegrafting for benign and malignant tumours*. J. Neurol. Neurosurg. Psychiatry 50: 151-154, 1987.

FINCHER E.F.: *Spontaneous subarachnoid haemorrage in intradural tumours of the lumbar sac. A clinical syndrome*. J. Neurosurg. 8: 576-584, 1951.

FINDLAY G.: *The role of vertebral body collapse in the management of malignant spinal cord compression*. J. Neurol. Neurosurg. Psychiatry 50: 151-154, 1987.

FINDLAY J., BERNSTEIN M., VANDERLINDEN R., RESCH L.: *Microsurgical resection of solitary intramedullary spinal cord metastases*. Neurosurgery 21: 911-915, 1987.

FINESCHI G.F.: *Importanza della diagnosi precoce nella cura chirurgica delle compressioni tumourali della cauda equina*. Arch. Putti 2: 267-282, 1952.

FIROOZNIA H., GOLIMBU C., RAFII M. ET AL.: *Computed tomography of spinal chordomas*. J. Comput. Tomogr. 10: 45-50, 1986.

FISCHER G., MANSUY L.: *Total removal of intramedullary ependymomas: follow-up study of 16 cases*. Surg. Neurol. 14: 243-249, 1980.

FLATLEY T.J., ANDERSON M.H., ANAST G.T.: *Spinal Instability due to malignant disease. Treatment by segmental spinal stabilization*. J. Bone Joint Surg. 66: 47-52, 1984.

FOERSTER O.: *A contribution to the study of the spinal gliomas of the spinal cord with special reference to their operability*. In: DAVIDENHOF N., *Livre jubilaire*, Leningrad, pp. 9-67, 1936.

FOKES E. JR, EARLE K.: *Ependymomas: clinical and pathological aspects*. J. Neurosurg. 30: 585-594, 1969.

FONTANA M., CARAPELLA C., CAROLI F., RICCIO A.: *Spinal meningioma: an unusual radiological and clinical case*. Neurosurgery 11: 811-812, 1982.

FORTUNA A., MOSCATELLI G.: *L'echinococco vertebrale*. Rivista di Neurologia 29: 762-767, 1959.

FORTUNA A.: *Epidermoide della cauda equina*. Il Lavoro Neuropsichiatrico 27: 479-491, 1960.

FORTUNA A., SILIPO P.: *Sugli angioreticulomi intramidollari*. Il Lavoro Neuropsichiatrico 29: 223-246, 1961.

FORTUNA A.: *Sindrome delle corna anteriori cervicali spondilogenetica.* Il Lavoro Neuropsichiatrico 29: 193-204, 1961.

FORTUNA A., SILIPO P.: *Sul valore diagnostico del fenomeno pseudomiotonico (di apertura della mano) nelle mielopatie da spondilosi cervicale.* Il Lavoro Neuropsichiatrico 29: 247-278, 1961.

FORTUNA A., RICCIO A.: *Un caso di ganglioneuroblastoma spinale a clessidra.* Il Policlinico 68: 1889-1894, 1961.

FORTUNA A., GUIDETTI B.: *Sugli angiomi vertebrali con compressione midollare.* Il Lavoro Neuropsichiatrico 29: 353-382, 1961.

FORTUNA A.: *Paraplegie acute da ernia del disco lombare: probabile patogenesi vascolare.* Il Lavoro Neuropsichiatrico 29: 481-518, 1961.

FORTUNA A.: *A proposito del valore diagnostico del fenomeno pseudomiotonico (di apertura della mano) nelle compressioni cervicali.* Il Lavoro Neuropsichiatrico 29: 393-400, 1961.

FORTUNA A., GIUFFRÈ R.: *Sintomatologia di Brown-Séquard nelle compressioni cervicali.* Il Lavoro Neuropsichiatrico 35: 569-580, 1962.

FORTUNA A., GUIDETTI B.: *Mielopatie vascolari. Trattato Italiano di Medicina Interna*, Prof. Paolo Introzzi, parte XII: 1212-1230, 1964.

FORTUNA A., LA TORRE E.: *Considerazioni su una sindrome di sezione trasversa midollare a $D_,$ evoluta a $D_,$ da aortografia translombare.* Rivista di Neurologia 36: 649-657, 1966.

FORTUNA A., LA TORRE E.: *Sindrome de section transversa por haemorragia en un neurinoma aspinal toracico.* Cienc. Neurol. 1: 13-14, 1967.

FORTUNA A., LA TORRE E.: *Un caso di mielopatia cervicale spondilogenetica con fibrillazione della lingua.* Minerva Neurochirurgica 11: 119-120, 1967.

FORTUNA A., SILIPO P.: *Quadro angiografico di un angioreticuloma midollare.* Nuntius Radiologicus 6: 713-718, 1967.

FORTUNA A., LA TORRE E.: *Neurinoma della cauda con emorragia subaracnoidea circoscritta.* Il Lavoro Neuropsichiatrico 43: 1-8, 1967.

FORTUNA A., SILIPO P.: *Prime esperienze con la flebografia cervicale transomatica nella diagnostica delle compressioni cervicali.* Minerva Neurochirurgica 13: 75-78, 1969.

FORTUNA A., GAMBACORTA D., OCCHIPINTI E.: *Spinal extradural meningiomas.* Neurochirurgia 12: 166-180, 1969.

FORTUNA A., LA TORRE E., OCCHIPINTI E.: *Le sciatiche spinali oncogenetiche.* Il Policlinico 77, fasc. 6: 1-11, 1970.

FORTUNA A., GIUFFRÈ R.: *Intramedullary glioblastoma.* Neurochirurgia 14: 14-23, 1971.

FORTUNA A., LA TORRE E., OCCHIPINTI E.: *The direction of blood flow in the cervical cord. An angiographic study of infants and children.* European Neurology 5: 335-342, 1971.

FORTUNA A., LA TORRE E.: *The lumbar root entrapment syndrome, with emphasis on clinical and myelographic findings.* European Neurology 16: 144-148, 1977.

FORTUNA A., LA TORRE E., CIAPPETTA P.: *Arachnoid diverticula: a unitary approach to spinal cysts communicating with the subarachnoid space.* Acta Neurochir. 39: 259-268, 1977.

FORTUNA A., PALMA L., MERCURI S.: *Spinal neuroepithelial cysts. Report of two cases and review of the literature.* Acta Neurochir. 45: 177-185, 1978.

FORTUNA A., CONTRATTI F., DI LORENZO N.: *Cervical intramedullary abscess extirpation by means of microsurgical techniques.* Journal Neurosurg. Sci. 23: 159-162, 1979.

FORTUNA A.: *Intraspinal disembryogenethic tumours in children (excluding dysraphism).* Phronesis 1: 91-95, 1980

FORTUNA A., CELLI P., PALMA L.: *Oligodendrogliomas of the spinal cord.* Acta Neurochir. 52: 305-329, 1980.

FORTUNA A., NOLLETTI A., NARDI P., CARUSO R.: *Spinal neurinomas and meningiomas in children.* Acta Neurochir. 55: 329-341, 1981.

FORTUNA A., GIUFFRÈ R., DI LORENZO N.: *Primary spinal tumours in infancy and childhood.* Zbl. Neurochirurgia 42: 87-98, 1981.

FORTUNA A., GIUFFRÈ R., DI LORENZO N.: *Cervical tumours of infancy and childhood.* J. of Neurosurg. Sciences 26, 259-264, 1981.

FORTUNA A.: *Chirurgia del midollo spinale.* Enciclopedia Medica Italiana: pp. 1405-1442, 1982.

FORTUNA A., MERCURI S.: *Intradural spinal cysts.* Acta Neurochir. 68: 289-314, 1983.

FORTUNA A., DI LORENZO N., NOLLETTI A., NARDI P.: *Solitary chondromas and osteochondro-*

mas of the spine provoking myeloradicular compression. Report on 6 cases treated surgically. Neurochirurgie 29: 271-278, 1983.

FORTUNA A.: *La sindrome precoce nei tumori spinali.* Conferenza all'Accademia Lancisiana di Roma, il 12 aprile 1994, Atti dell'Accademia Lancisiana, 38: 64-69.

FOX M., ONOFRIO B.: *The natural history and management of symptomatic and asymptomatic vertebral haemangiomas.* J. Neurosurg. 78: 36-45, 1993.

FRASER R., PATERSON D., SIMPSON D.: *Orthopedic aspects of spinal tumours in children.* J. Bone Joint Surg. 59: 143-151, 1977.

FREIDBERG SR: *Removal of an ossified ventral thoracic meningioma. Case report.* J. Neurosurg. 37: 728-730, 1972.

FRIED H., SKRZYPCZAK J., HOHREIN D.: *Spinal gliomas including ependymomas.* Zentralbl. Neurochir. 49: 273-275, 1988.

FRIEDMAN W.: *Somatosensory evoked potentials.* In: Clinical Neurosurgery 34: 187-238, 1986.

FRIEDMAN D., TARTAGLINO L., FLANDERS A.: *Intradural schwannomas of the spine: MR findings with emphasis on contrast enhancement characteristics.* AJR 158: 1347-1350, 1992.

FRIEDMAN D., FLANDERS A., TARTAGLINO L.: *Vascular neoplasms and malformations, ischemia, and haemorrhage affecting the spinal cord: MR imaging findings.* AJR 162: 685-692, 1994.

FRUGONI P., IRACI G., COSTANTINI E. ET AL.: *Considerazioni su 43 casi di tumori intrarachidei operati d'urgenza.* Minerva Neuroch. 11: 75-83, 1967.

GAGLIARDI F., GAMBACORTA D.: *Su di un caso di angiolipoma dorsale epidurale.* Gaz. Internaz. Med. Chir. (Roma) 73: 5602-5608, 1968.

GARCIA PICAZO A., CAPILLA RAMIREZ P., PULIDO RIVAS-P., GARCIA DE SOLA R.: *Utility of surgery in the treatment of epidural vertebral metastases.* Acta Neurochir. 103: 131-138, 1990.

GARFINKLE W., YUDD A.: *Calcified intraspinal meningioma detected by computed tomography.* Comput. Radiol. 6: 305-307, 1982.

GARRIDO E., STEIN B.: *Microsurgical removal of intramedullary spinal cord tumours.* Surg. Neurol. 7: 215-219, 1977.

GARZA MERCADO R.: *Diastematomyelia and intramedullary epidermoid spinal cord tumour combined with extradural teratoma in an adult.* J. Neurosurg. 58: 954-958, 1983.

GASTON A., LAREDO J.D., ASSOULINE E.: *Compressive vertebral haemangiomas. Value of imaging for diagnosis and definition of treatment.* Neurochirurgie 35: 275-283, 1989.

GAUTIER-SMITH P.C.: *Clinical aspect of spinal neurofibromas.* Brain 90: 359-394, 1967.

GEORGE B., LAURIAN C., KERAVEL Y., COPHIGNON J.: *Extradural and hourglass cervical neurinomas: the vertebral artery problem.* Neurosurgery 16: 591-594, 1985.

GIUFFRÈ R.: *Intradural spinal lipomas. Review of the literature (99 cases) and report of an additional case.* Acta Neurochir. 14: 69-95, 1966.

GIUFFRÈ R., GAMBACORTA D.: *Lipoma of the spinal cord. Case report.* J. Neurosurg. 35: 335-337, 1971.

GIUFFRÈ R.: *Spinal lipomas.* In: VINKEN P.J., BRUYN G.W. (eds), *Handbook Of Clinical Neurology,* vol. 20: "Tumours Of The Spine And Spinal Cord", part 11 North Holland, Amsterdam, pp. 389-414, 1976.

GIUFFRÈ R., DI LORENZO N., FORTUNA A.: *Cervical tumours of infancy and childhood.* J. Neurosurg. Sci. 25: 259-264, 1981.

GOODRICH A., WOLF C., ALLEN M. JR: *Intradural dermoid cyst. A case report.* Spine 9: 832-834, 1984.

GORMAN P., RIGAMONTI D., JOSLYN J.: *Intramedullary and extramedullary schwannoma of the cervical spinal cord case report.* Surg. Neurol. 32: 459-462 1989.

GOY A., PINTO R., RAGHAVENDRA B., EPSTEIN F.J., KRICHEFF I.: *Intramedullary spinal cord tumours: MR imaging, with emphasis on associated cyst.* Radiology 161: 381-386, 1986.

GRANIERI U., MAIURI F., COLANTUONO C., MAIURI L.: *Vertebral osteoid osteoma, a rare cause of root compression and scoliosis in children.* Riv. Neurol. 50: 278-284, 1980.

GRANT F., AUSTIN G.: *The diagnosis, treatment, and prognosis of tumours affecting the spinal cord in children.* J. Neurosurg. 13: 535-545, 1956.

GRAWE A., SIEDSCHLAG W.D., NISCH G.: *Metastases of the spinal canal clinic and results of operation.* Zentralbl. Neurochir. 49: 340-343, 1988.

GREENWOOD J. JR: *Intramedullary tumours of the spinal cord. A follow-up study after total surgical removal.* J. Neurosurg. 20: 665-668, 1963.

GREENWOOD J.: *Surgical removal of intramedullary tumours.* J. Neurosurg. 26: 276-282, 1967.

GREM J.L., BURGESS J., TRUMP D.: *Clinical features and natural history of intramedullary spinal cord metastasis.* Cancer 56: 2305-2314, 1985.

GRIEBEL R.W., KHAN M., ROZDILSKY B.: *Spinal extradural angiolipoma. A case report and literature review.* Spine 11: 47-48, 1986.

GRISOLD W., PERNETZKY G., JELLINGER K.: *Giant cell glioblastoma of the thoracic cord.* Acta Neurochir. 58: 121-126, 1981.

GROSSMAN S.A., WEISSMAN D.E., WANG H. ET AL.: *Early diagnosis of spinal epidural metastases using out-patient computed tomographic myelography.* Eur. J. Cancer 26: 495-499, 1990.

GUHA A., RESCH L., TATOR C.: *Subependymoma of the thoracolumbar cord. Case report.* J. Neurosurg. 71: 781-787, 1989.

GUIDETTI B., CARLONI G.: *Tumori spinali.* Riv. di Pat. Nerv. e Ment. 76: 1-34, 1955.

GUIDETTI B.: *Mielopatie da spondilosi cervicale.* Bologna Med. Ed., p. 245, 1958.

GUIDETTI B., FORTUNA A., MOSCATELLI G., RICCIO A.: *I tumori intramidollari.* Lav. Neuropsichiat. 35: 1-409, 1964.

GUIDETTI B., FORTUNA A.: *Trattamento conservativo e chirurgico delle Mielopatie da Discoartrosi.* Atti del XVI Congresso Nazionale di Neurologia, vol. 1, pp, 181-231, Pensiero Scientifico Editore, 1967.

GUIDETTI B., FORTUNA A.: *Surgical treatment of intramedullary haemangioblastomas of spinal cord: report of six cases.* J. Neurosurg. 27: 530-540, 1967.

GUIDETTI B.: *Intramedullary tumours of the spinal cord.* Acta Neuroch. 17: 7-23, 1967.

GUIDETTI B., FORTUNA A.: *Long term result of surgical treatment of myelopathy due to cervical spondylosis.* J. Neurosurgery 30: 714-721, 1969.

GUIDETTI B.: *Removal of extramedullary benign spinal cord tumours.* Advances and Technical Standard in Neurosurgery, vol. 1: 173-197, 1974; Springer-Verlag, Wien-New York.

GUIDETTI B., FORTUNA A.: *Differential diagnosis of intramedullary and extramedullary tumours.* In: VINKEN P.J., BRUYN G.W. (eds), *Handbook of Clinical Neurology Amsterdam*, North-Holland, vol. 19, pp. 51-75, 1975.

GUIDETTI B., GAGLIARDI F.M.: *Epidermoid and dermoid cysts. Clinical evaluation and late surgical results.* J. Neurosurg. 47: 12-18, 1977.

GUIDETTI B., FORTUNA A., ZAMPONI C., LUNARDI P.: *Cervical spondylosis myelopathy.* Advances in Neurosurgery N8, Springer-Verlag, Berlin-New York, pp. 104-111, 1980.

GUIDETTI B., SPALLONE A.: *Benign extramedullary tumours of the foramen magnum.* Surg. Neurol. 13: 9-17, 1980.

GUIDETTI B., MERCURI S., VAGNOZZI R.: *Long-term results of the surgical treatment of 129 intramedullary spinal gliomas.* J. Neurosurg. 54: 323-330, 1981.

GUIDETTI B., SPALLONE A.: *Benign extramedullary tumours of the foramen magnum.* Advances and Technical Standard in Neurosurgery, vol. 16: 83-120, 1988; Springer-Verlag, Wien-New York.

HADDAD FS., ABLA A., ALLAM C.K.: *Extradural spinal angiolipoma.* Surg. Neurol. 26: 473-486, 1986.

HADLEY M., SONNTAG V., AMOS M. ET AL.: *Three-dimensional computed tomography in the diagnosis of vertebral column pathological conditions.* Neurosurgery 21: 186-192, 1987.

HAFT H., RANSOHOFF J., CARTER S.: *Spinal cord tumours in children.* Pediatrics 23: 1152-1159, 1959.

HAFT H., SHENKIN H.: *Spinal epidural meningioma. Case report.* J. Neurosurg. 20: 801-804, 1963.

HALL A.J., MACKAY N.S.: *The results of laminectomy for compression of the cord or cauda equina by extradural malignant tumours.* J. Bone Joint Surg. 55: 497-505, 1973.

HAMBY W.: *Tumours in the spinal canal in childhood.* J. Neuropath. Exper. Neurol. 3: 397-343, 1944.

HANAKITA J., SUWA H., NAGAYASU S. ET AL.: *Clinical features of intradural neurinomas in the cauda equina and around the conus medullaris.* Neurochirurgia 35: 145-149, 1992.

HARDISON H.D., PACKER R.J., RORKE L.B. ET AL.: *Outcome of children with primary intramedullary spinal cord tumours.* Childs Nerv. Syst. 3: 89-92, 1987.

HARKEY H.L., CROCKARD A.: *Spinal meningiomas: clinical features.* In: AL MEFTY O., *Meningiomas*, pp. 593-601, Raven Press, New York, 1991.

HARRINGTON K.: *Anterior cord decompression and spinal stabilization for patients with metastatic lesions of the spine.* J. Neurosurg. 61: 107-117, 1984.

HAUGHT O, POJUNAS K. ET AL.: *Differentiation of intramedullary neoplasm and cysts by MRI.* AJR 149: 159-164, 1987.

HAUTZER NW., AIYESIMOJU A., ROBITAILLE Y.: *"Primary" spinal intramedullary lymphomas: a review.* Ann. Neurol. 14: 62-66, 1983.

HEALY M., HERZ D.A., PEARL L.: *Spinal haemangioma.* Neurosurgery 13: 689-691, 1983.

HELWEG LARSEN S., SORENSEN P.: *Symptoms and signs in metastatic spinal cord compression: a study of progression from first symptom until diagnosis in 153 patients.* Eur. J. Cancer 30a: 396-398, 1994.

HENDRICK E.: *Spinal cord tumours in children.* In: YOUMANS JR: *Neurological Surgery*, vol. 4, 2nd ed., Saunders, Philadelphia, pp. 3215-3222, 1982.

HERB E., SCHWACHENWALD R., NOWAK G., MULLER H., REUSCHE E.: *Acute bleeding into a filum terminale ependymoma.* Neurosurg. Rev 13: 243-245, 1990.

HERMAN SD., MERGARZADEH M., BONAKDARPOUR A., DALINKA M.: *The role of Magnetic Resonance Imaging in giant cell tumour of the bone.* Skeletal Radiol. 16: 635-643, 1987.

HERRMANN H.D., NEUSS M., WINKLER D.: *Intramedullary spinal cord tumours resected with CO_2 laser microsurgical technique: recent experience in fifteen patients.* Neurosurgery 22: 518-522, 1988.

HIDA K., IWASAKI Y., CHO K., IMAMURA H., ABE H.: *Gliomas of the conus medullaris.* Paraplegia 32: 52-58, 1994.

HILDEBRANDT G., ZIERSKI J., CHRISTOPHIS ET AL.: *Giant cell tumours, aneurysmatic bone cysts and osteoid osteomas of the vetebral column.* Neurochirurgia 31: 107-113 1988.

HILL M., RICHARDS M., GREGORY W. ET AL.: *Spinal cord compression in breast cancer: a review of 70 cases.* Br. J. Cancer 68: 969-973, 1993.

HIRANO H., SUZUKI H., SAKAKIBARA T. ET AL.: *Foramen magnum and upper cervical cord tumours. Diagnostic problems.* Clin. Orthop. 176: 171-177, 1983.

HODGE C., JONES M.: *Syringomyelia and spinal cord tumours.* Curr. Opin Neurol. Neurosurg. 4: 597-600, 1991.

HOFFMAN G., WARAT P., GALIBERT P., MEIGNIE S., LAINE M.E.: *Lipomes intra medullaires de la region cervico dorsale.* Rev. Neurol. 103: 558-567, 1981.

HOUTTEVILLE J., DECROIX J., HURTH M.: *A slowly progressive disorder of the spinal cord in a young woman.* Rev. Neurol. Paris 143: 698-705, 1987.

HURT M.: *Les haemangioblastomes intrarachidiens.* Neurochirurgie 21: 1-136, 1975.

HOVE B., GYLDENSTED C.: *Spiculated vertebral metastases from prostatic carcinoma. Report of first two cases.* Neuroradiology 32: 337-339, 1990.

HU HP., HUANG Q.L.: *Signal intensity correlation of MRI with pathological findings in spinal neurinomas.* Neuroradiol. 34: 98-102, 1992.

HUDDART R., TRAISH D., ASHLEY S. ET AL.: *Management of spinal astrocytoma with conservative surgery and radiotherapy.* Br. J. Neurosurg. 7: 473-481, 1993.

HULSHOF M.C., MENTEN J., DITO J.J. ET AL.: *Treatment results in primary intraspinal gliomas.* Radiother. Oncol. 29: 294-300, 1993.

HUOS A.G.: *Bone tumours: diagnosis treatment and prognosis.* Philadelphia, WB Saunders Co., 1979.

IOB I., ANDRIOLI G.C., RIGOBELLO L., SALAR G.: *An unusual onset of a spinal cord tumour: subarachnoid bleeding and papilloedema. Case report.* Neurochirurgia (Stuttg.), 23: 112-116, 1980.

IRACI G., PESERICO L., SALAR G.: *Intraspinal neuromas and meningiomas.* Int. Surg. 56: 289-303, 1971.

ISHII N., MATSUZAWA H., HOUKIN K.: *An evaluation of 70 spinal schwannomas using conventional Computed Tomography and Magnetic Resonance Imaging.* Neuroradiol. 33: 542, 1991.

JAMES H., WILLIAMS J., BROCK W. ET AL.: *Radical removal of lipomas of the conus and cauda equina with laser microneurosurgery.* Neurosurgery 15: 340-343, 1984.

JANIN Y., EPSTEIN J., CARRAS R., KHAN A.: *Osteoid osteomas and osteoblastomas of the spine.* Neurosurgery 8: 31-38, 1981.

JOHNSTON F., UTTLEY D., MARSH H.: *Synchronous vertebral decompression and posterior stabilization in the treatment of spinal malignancy.* Neurosurgery 25: 872-876, 1989.

JRASEK A.: *Diagnosis and treatment of intraspinal tumours.* IX Congr. Int. Chir., Madrid, 667-719, 1932.

KAK V., PRABHAKAR S., KHOSLA V., BANERJEE A.: *Solitary osteochondroma of spine causing spinal cord compression.* Clin. Neurol. Neurosurg. 87: 135-138, 1985.

KARIAN J., DEFILIPP. G., BUCHHEIT W.A. ET AL.: *Vertebral osteochondroma causing spinal cord compression: case report.* Neurosurgery 14: 483-484, 1984.

KARGER P.: *Die Wurzelschmerzen bei intramedullaren Neubildungen.* Monatschr. F. Psych. Neurol. 39: 167-178, 1916.

KATZ K., REICHENTAL E., ISRAELI J.: *Surgical treatment of spinal meningiomas.* Neurochirurgia 24: 21-22, 1981.

KAUFMAN B., PARK T.: *Congenital spinal cord astrocytomas.* Child's Nerv. Syst. 8: 389-393, 1992.

KAWAKAMI N., MIMATSU K., KATO F.: *Intraoperative sonography of intramedullary spinal cord tumours.* Neuroradiology 34: 436-439, 1992.

KAYA U., OZDEN B., TURANTAN M.I. ET AL.: *Spinal epidural meningioma in childhood: a case report.* Neurosurgery 10: 746-747, 1982.

KENDRICK F., BONNIN J., GARCIA J.: *Metastases of a spinal glioblastoma multiforme into an intracranial arachnoid cyst.* Neurosurgery 20: 780-783, 1987.

KERNHOAN J., WOLTMAN H., ADSON A.: *Intramedullary tumours of the spinal cord. A review of fifty-one cases, with an attempt at histological classification.* Arch. Neurol. Psych. 29: 287-305, 1931.

KIM R., SPENCER S., MEREDITH R. ET AL.: *Extradural spinal cord compression: analysis of factors determining functional prognosis prospective study.* Radiology 176: 279-282, 1990.

KORMOS R., TUCKER W., BILBAO J. ET AL.: *Subarachnoid haemorrhage due to a spinal cord haemangioblastoma: case report.* Neurosurgery 6: 657-660, 1980.

KOSTUIK J., ERRICO T., GLEASON T.F. ET AL.: *Spinal stabilization of vertebral column tumours.* Spine 13: 250-256, 1988.

KROL G., SUNDARESAN N., DECK M.: *Computed tomography of axial chordomas.* J. Comput. Asst. Tomogr. 7: 286-289, 1983.

KULALI A., VON WILD K., HOBIK H.: *Subarachnoid haemorrhage with acute cauda symptom due to spinal tumour.* Neurochirurgia 32: 87-90, 1989.

KUMAR S., GULATI D., MANN K.: *Intraspinal dermoids.* Neurochirurgia (Stuttg.) 20: 105-108, 1977.

KUMAR S., KAZA R.C., MAITRA T.K., CHANDRA M.: *Extradural spinal meningioma arising from a nerve root: case report.* J. Neurosurg. 52: 728-729, 1980.

KURODA S., ABE H., AKINO M. ET AL.: *Infiltrating spinal angiolipoma causing myelopathy: case report.* Neurosurgery 27: 315-318, 1990.

LANTOS G., EPSTEIN F., KORY L.: *Magnetic resonance imaging of intradural spinal lipoma.* Neurosurgery 20: 469-472, 1987.

LAREDO J.D., ASSOULINE E., GASTON A. ET AL.: *Evaluation radiologique de l'activité des hèmangiomes vertebraux isolés.* Neurochirurgie 35: 284-288, 1989.

LAUBICHLER W.: *Spinale Geschwulste in pädiatrischler Neurochirurgie.* Stuttgard, Georg Thieme Verlag, pp. 647-662, 1967.

LESOIN F., FRANZ K., VILLETTE L. ET AL.: *Usefulness of the bilateral anterolateral approach in operations on the cervical spine.* Surg. Neurol. 27: 228-232, 1987.

LEONARDI M., RUFFATO C., KUNERT A.: *TC e RMN della colonna lombare e del midollo spinale.* Summa Radiografica, Piccin, Padova, 1988.

LEVY W. JR, BAY J., DOHN D.: *Spinal cord meningioma.* J. Neurosurg. 57: 804-812, 1982.

LEVY W.: *The electrophysiological monitoring of motor pathways.* Clinic Neurosurgery 34: 239-260, 1986.

LI M., LARSSON E.: *MR imaging of intradural extramedullary tumours.* Acta Radiol. 33: 207-212, 1992.

LIEN H., BLOMLIE V., HEIMDAL K.: *Magnetic resonance imaging of malignant extradural tumours with acute spinal cord compression*. Acta Radiol. 31: 187-190, 1990.

LIM V., SOBEL D.F., ZYROFF J.: *Spinal cord pial metastases: MR imaging with gadopetetate dimeglumine*. AJNR 11: 975-982, 1990.

LINDGREN E.: *Roentgenologie einschliesslich Kontrastmethoden*. In: OLIVECRONA H., TONNIS W (eds), *Handbuch der Neurochirurgie*, vol. II, Berlin, Springer, 1954.

LINKOWSKI G., TSAI F., RECHER L. ET AL.: *Solitary osteochondroma with spinal cord compression*. Surg. Neurol. 23: 388-390, 1985.

LIST C.: *Intraspinal epidermoids, dermoids and dermal sinuses*. Surg. Gynecol. Obstet. 73: 525-538, 1941.

LODRINI S., LASIO G., CIMINO C., PLUCHINO F.: *Haemangioblastoma: clinical characteristics, surgical results and immunohistochemical studies*. J. Neurosurg. Sci. 35: 179-185, 1991.

LOFTUS C., ROZARIO R., PRAGER R., SCOTT R.: *Solitary osteochondroma of T4 with thoracic cord compression*. Surg. Neurol. 13: 355-357, 1980.

LONG D.M.: *Vascular ultrastructure in human meningiomas and schwannomas*. J. Neurosurg. 38: 409-419, 1973.

LOVE J.: *The differential diagnosis of intraspinal tumours and protruded intervertebral disks and their surgical treatment*. J. Neurosurg. 1: 275-290, 1944.

LOVE J., THELEN E.P., DODGE H.W. JR: *Tumours of the foramen magnum*. J. Int. Coll. Surg. 22: 1-77, 1954.

LUCANTONI D., TASSI G., MAGLIANI V. ET AL.: *Osteochondroma of the cervical spine: a rare case of cervical radiculopathy*. Riv. Neurobiol. 38: 73-76 1992.

LUNARDI P., MISSORI P., GAGLIARDI F.M., FORTUNA A.: *Long term results of the surgical treatment of spinal dermoid and epidermoid tumours*. Neurosurgery 25: 860-864, 1989.

LUNARDI P., MISSORI P., FERRANTE L., FORTUNA A.: *Long term results of surgical treatment of spinal lipomas*. Acta Neurochirurgica 104: 64-68, 1990.

LUNARDI P., MISSORI P., FRANCO C., DELFINI R., FORTUNA A.: *Hard rock spinal meningioma. Case report and revue of the literature*. J. Neurosurg. Sci. 36: 243-246, 1992.

LUNARDI P., CERVONI L., MALECI A., FORTUNA A.: *A isolated haemangioblastoma of spinal cord: report of 18 cases and review of the literature*. Acta Neurochirurgica 122: 236-239, 1993.

LUNARDI P., LICASTRO G., MISSORI P., FERRANTE L., FORTUNA A.: *Management of intramedullary tumours in children*. Acta Neurochirurgica 120: 59-65, 1993.

LYONS M., O'NEIL B., MARSH R., KURTIN P.: *Primary spinal epidural non Hodgkin's lymphoma: report of eight patients and review of the literature*. Neurosurgery 30: 675-680, 1992.

MAHMOOD A., CACCAMO D., MORGAN J.: *Tenosynovial giant cell tumour of the cervical spine. Case report*. J. Neurosurg. 77: 952-955, 1992.

MAIURI F., SIGNORELLI C., GAMBARDELLA A. ET AL.: *Osteoid osteomas of the spine*. Surg. Neurol. 25: 375-380, 1986.

MAIURI F., D'ANDREA F.: *Neurochirurgia*, 2nd ed. Editoriale Bios, p. 656, 1992.

MALBRAIN M.L., KAMPER A.M., LAMBRECHT G.L. ET AL.: *Filum terminale ependymoma revealed by acute cauda equina compression syndrome following intratumoral and spinal subarachnoid haemorrhage in a patient on oral anticoagulants*. Acta Neurol. Belg. 94: 35-43, 1994.

MALIK G., TOMECEK E., SCHMIDEK H. ET AL.: *Spinal meningiomas*. In: *Meningiomas and their surgical management*, edited by H.H. Schmidek, pp. 483-489, WB Saunders Co., Philadelphia, 1991.

MALIS L.: *Intramedullary spinal cord tumours*. Clin. Neurosurg. 25: 512-539, 1978.

MANABE S., TATEISHI A., ABE M., OHNO T.: *Surgical treatment of metastatic tumours of the spine*. Spine 14: 41-47, 1989.

MANNO N., UIHLEIN A., KERNOHAN J.: *Intraspinal epidermoids*. J. Neurosurg. 19: 754-765, 1962.

MARCHESI D., BOOS N., AEBI M.: *Surgical treatment of tumours of the cervical spine and first two thoracic vertebrae*. J. Spinal Disord. 6: 489-496, 1993.

MARSH B., BONFIGLIO M., BRADY L., ENNEKING W.: *Benign osteoblastoma: range of manifestations*. J. Bone Joint Surg. 57A: 1-9, 1975.

MARSH H.: *Metastatic disease of the spine*. Br. J. Neurosurg. 4: 167-170, 1990.

MARTINEZ LAGE J., MASEGOAS J., SOLA J., POZA M.: *Epidermoid cyst occurring within a lumbosacral myelomeningocele.* J. Neurosurg. 59: 1095-1097, 1983.

MASCALCHI M., ARNETOLI G., DAL POZZO G. ET AL.: *Spinal epidural angiolipoma: MR findings.* Am. J. Neuroradiol. 12: 744-745, 1991.

MASSARE C.L.: *Rachis et moelle. L'imagerie, aujourdhui.* Vigot, Paris, 1988.

MASTRONARDI L., FERRANTE L., SCARPINATI M., GAGLIARDI F.M., CELLI P., FORTUNA A.: *Intradural extramedullary cavernous angioma. A case report.* Neurosurgery 29: 900-902, 1991.

MATSON D.D., TACHDJIAN M.: *Intraspinal tumours in infants and children. Review of 115 cases.* Postgrad Med. 34: 279-285, 1963.

MATSON D.D.: *Neurosurgery of infancy and childhood.* Springfield, Charles C. Thomas, 2nd ed., 1969.

MATSUMOTO S., HASUO K., UCHINO A. ET AL.: *MRI of intradural extramedullary spinal neurinomas and meningiomas.* Clin. Imaging 17: 46-52, 1993.

MATSUSHIAMA K., SHINOHARA Y., YAMAMOTO M. ET AL.: *Spinal extradural angiolipoma: MR and CT diagnosis.* J. Comput. Assisted Tomography 11: 1104-1106, 1987.

MATSUZAKI H., TOKUHASHI Y., WAKABAYASHI K., TORIYAMA S.: *Clinical values of intraoperative ultrasonography for spinal tumours.* Spine 17: 1392-1399, 1992.

MAUSER H., DOKKUM T.: *Astrocytomas involving the whole spinal cord. Two case reports.* Clin. Neurol. Neurosurg. 83: 239-245, 1981.

MCAFEE P., ZDEBLICK T.: *Tumours of the thoracic and lumbar spine: surgical treatment via the anterior approach.* J. Spinal Disord. 2: 145-154, 1989.

MCCORMICK P.C., TORRES R., POST K.: *Intramedullary ependymomas of spinal cord.* J. Neurosurgery 72: 523-533, 1990.

MCCORMICK P.C.: *Anatomic principles of intradural spinal surgery.* Clinical Neurosurgery 41: 204-223, 1993.

MCCORMICK P., TORRES R., POST K., STEIN B.: *Intramedullary ependymoma of the spinal cord.* J. Neurosurg. 72: 523-532, 1986.

MCGILLICUDDY G., SHUCART W., KWAN E.: *Intradural spinal lipomas.* Neurosurgery 21: 343-346, 1987.

MCCULLOCK A.: *Principles of microsurgery for lumbar disc disease,* p. 40, Raven Press, New York, 1989.

MEMON M.Y., SCHNECK L.: *Ventral spinal tumour: the value of computed tomography in its localization.* Neurosurgery 8: 108-111, 1981.

MENDELSSON R.A., MORA F.: *Spontaneous subarachnoid haemorrage caused by ependymoma of the filum terminale.* J. Neurosurgery 15: 460-463, 1958.

MICHILLI R., TZONOS P., IGLESIAS ROZAS JR: *Spinal extradural angiolipoma: case report and literature review.* Neurochirurgia 36: 63-65, 1993.

MIGLIAVACCA F.: *Surgery of primary and metastatic spinal cord tumours.* Minerva Med. 75: 1355-1357, 1984.

MILZ H., HAMER J.: *Extradural spinal meningiomas. Report of two cases.* Neurochirurgia 26: 126-129, 1983.

MOFFIE D., STEFANKO S.: *Intramedullary metastasis.* Clin. Neurol. Neurosurg. 82: 199-202, 1980.

MOHASSEB G.: *Intraspinal dermoid cyst communicating with a dermal sinus.* Neurol. India 17: 16-21, 1969.

MORI K., KAMIMURA Y., UCHIDA Y. ET AL.: *Large intramedullary lipoma of the cervical cord and posterior fossa. Case report.* J. Neurosurg. 64: 974-976, 1986.

MORIWAKA F., HOZEN H., NAKANE K. ET AL.: *Myelopathy due to osteochondroma: MR and CT studies.* J. Comput. Assisted Tomography 14: 128-130, 1990.

MORK SJ., LOKEN A.: *Ependymoma. A follow-up study of 101 cases.* Cancer 40: 907-913, 1977.

MOSCATELLI G., SILIPO P.: *Su un caso di lipoma midollare sottodurale.* Riv. Neurol. 31: 274-286, 1961.

MOTOMOCHI M., MAKITA Y., NABESHIMA S., AOYAMA I.: *Spinal epidural meningioma in childhood.* Surg. Neurol. 13: 5-7, 1980.

MUROTA T., SYMON L.: *Surgical management of haemangioblastoma of the spinal cord: a report of 18 cases.* Neurosurgery 25: 699-708, 1989.

MYLES S.T., MACRAE M.E.: *Benign osteoblastoma of the spine in childhood.* J. Neurosurg. 68: 884-888, 1988.

NAIDU M.R.C., DINAKER L.: *Intramedullary mass lesions of the spinal cord.* Clin. Neurol. Neurosurg. 91: 135-138, 1989.

NASSAR S.I., CORRELL J.W.: *Subarachnoid haemorrhage due to spinal cord tumours.* Neurology 18: 87-94, 1968.

NEMOTO O., MOSER R. JR, VAN DAM B.: *Osteoblastoma of the spine: a review of 75 cases.* Spine 15: 1272-1280, 1990.

NEMOTO Y., INOUE Y., TASHIRO T. ET AL.: *Intramedullary spinal cord tumours: significance of associated haemorrhage at MR imaging.* Radiology 182: 793-796, 1992.

NEUMANN H.P.H., EGGERT H.R., WEIGEL K. ET AL.: *Haemangioblastomas of the central nervous system. A 10 year study with special reference to von Hippel Lindau syndrome.* J. Neurosurg. 70: 24-30, 1989.

NEWTON T.H., POTTS D.G.: *Computed tomography of the spine and spinal cord.* Clavadel Press, U.S.A. San Anselmo, pp. 1-413, 1983.

NGUYEN J.D., DJINDJIAN M., BADIANE S.: *Vertebral haemangiomas with neurologic symptoms. Clinical presentation: results of the Société Française de Neurochirurgie series.* Neurochirurgie 35: 270-274, 1989.

NISHIO S., FUKUI M., KITAMURA K., NUMAGUCHI Y.: *Intraspinal meningioma in childhood.* Child's Brain 8: 382 389, 1981.

NITTNER M.: *Spinal meningiomas, neurinomas and neurofibromas and hourglass tumours.* In: VINKEN P.J., BRUYN G.W. (eds): *Handbook of Clinical Neurology,* Amsterdam, North-Holland, vol. 20, pp. 177-322, 1976.

NOSTROM C.W., KERNHOAN W.J., LOVE J.L.: *One hundred primary caudal tumours.* J. Amer. Med. Ass. 178: 1071-1077, 1961.

O'CONNOR G., ROBERTS T.: *Spinal cord compression by an osteochondroma in a patient with multiple osteochondromatosis. Case report.* J. Neurosurg. 60: 420-423, 1984.

ODDSSON B.: *Spinal meningioma.* Copenhagen, E. Munksgaard, 1947.

OJEMANN R.: *Management of cranial and spinal meningiomas (honored guest presentation).* Clin. Neurosurg. 40: 321 383, 1993.

OKAWARA S.: *Ruptured spinal ependymoma simulating bacterial meningitis.* Arch. Neurol. 40: 54 55, 1983.

O'ROURKE T., GEORGE C., REDMOND J. ET AL.: *Spinal computed tomography and computed tomographic metrizamide myelography in the early diagnosis of metastatic disease.* J. Clin. Oncol. 4: 576-583, 1986.

OSBORN A.G.: *Tumours, cysts and tumorlike lesions of the spine and spinal cord.* In: *Osborn AG Diagnostic Neuroradiology,* Mosby ed., pp. 876-916, 1994.

OTSUBO H., HOFFMAN H., HUMPHREYS R. ET AL.: *Detection and management of gangliogliomas in children.* Surg. Neurol. 38: 371 378, 1992.

PAGNI C.A., FACCANI G., LANOTTE M.: *I tumori primitivi del midollo spinale. Progressi di diagnosi e terapia.* Ed. Minerva Medica, Torino, 1981.

PAGNI C.A.: *I meningiomi spinali.* CIC Edizioni Internazionali, pp. 1-249, 1989.

PAGNI C.A., CANAVERO S., RIEDEL C., APUZZO M.: *Spinal epidural angiolipoma: rare or unreported?* Neurosurgery 31: 758-764, 1992.

PAILLAS J., SERRATRICE G., LEGRÈ J.: *Les tumeurs primitives du rachis.* Paris, Masson, 1963.

PALKOVIC S., WASSMANN H., BONSE R., KASHAB M.: *Angiolipoma of the spinal cord. Magnetic resonance imaging and microsurgical management.* Surg. Neurol. 29: 243-245, 1988.

PALMER F., BLUM P.: *Osteochondroma with spinal cord compression. Report of three cases.* J. Neurosurg. 52: 842-845, 1980.

PANSINI A., CONTI P.: *On some rare spreading cervical lesions.* J. Neurosurg. Sci. 25: 255-257, 1981.

PANSINI A.: *Diagnostica precoce delle compressioni mieloradicolari; Rx, TC, RM.* Piccin Editore, Padova, p. 204, 1987.

PANSINI A., LO RE F., CONTI P., DE LUCA G. ET AL.: *Surgical treatment of posttraumatic osteochondroma at D11 D12 with ultrasonic osteotome.* Riv. Neuroradiologia 6: 231-238, 1993.

PARENTI G., FIORI L., MARCONI F., TUSINI G.: *Primary cauda equina tumours.* J. Neurosurg. Sciences 37: 149-156, 1993.

PARIZEL P., BALERIAUX D., RODESCH G. ET AL.: *Gd-Dtpa-Enhanced MR imaging of spinal tumours.* Am. J. Neuroradiol. 10: 249-258, 1989.

PATRONAS N., BROWN F., DUDA E.: *Multiple meningiomas in the spinal canal.* Surg. Neurol. 13: 78-80, 1980.

PERRIN R., LIVINGSTON K., AARABI B.: *Intradural extramedullary spinal metastasis. A report of 10 cases.* J. Neurosurg. 56: 835-837, 1982.

PIERRE KAHN A., LACOMBE J., PICHON J. ET AL.: *Intraspinal lipomas with spina bifida. Prognosis and treatment in 73 cases.* J. Neurosurg. 65: 756-761, 1986.

PISTOLESI G.F., BERGAMO ANDREIS I.A.: *L'immagine diagnostica del rachide.* Ed. Libreria Cortina, Verona, p. 748, 1987.

POOL J.: *The surgery of the spinal cord tumours.* Clin. Neurosurg. 17: 310-330, 1970.

POPPE E., LIVERUD K., EFKIND J.: *Osteosarcoma.* Acta Chir. Scand. 134: 549-556, 1968.

PORTENOY R., GALER B., SALAMON O. ET AL.: *Identification of epidural neoplasm. Radiography and bone scintigraphy in the symptomatic and asymptomatic spine.* Cancer 64: 2207-2213, 1989.

POST K., STEIN B.: *Surgical management of spinal cord tumours and arteriovenous malformations.* In: SCHMIDEK H.H., SWEET W.H. (eds), *Operative Neurosurgical Techniques, Indications, Methods, And Results,* vol. 2, Grune And Stratton, New York, pp. 1445-1476, 1988.

PREUL M.C., LEBLANC R., TAMPIERI D. ET AL.: *Spinal angiolipomas. Report of three cases.* J. Neurosurg. 78: 280-286, 1993.

PRIETO A., CANTU R.C.: *Spinal subarachnoid haemorrhage associated with neurofibroma of the cauda equina.* J. Neurosurg. 27: 63-69, 1967.

PRITZ M.: *Evaluation and treatment of intradural tumours located anterior to the cervicomedullary junction by a lateral suboccipital approach.* Acta Neurochir. 113: 74-81, 1991.

PULJIC S., SCHECHTER M.: *Multiple spinal canal meningiomas.* AJNR 1: 325-327, 1980.

PUNT J., PRITCHARD J., PINCOTT JR, TILL K.: *Neuroblastoma: a review of 21 cases presenting with spinal cord compression.* Cancer 45: 3095-3101, 1980.

RAGHAVENDRA B., EPSTEIN F., McCLEARY L.: *Intramedullary spinal cord in children: localization by intra operative sonography.* AJNR 5: 395-397, 1984.

RAIMONDI A.J., GUTIERREZ F., DI ROCCO C.: *Laminotomy and total reconstruction of the spinal arch for spinal canal surgery in childhood.* J. Neurosurg. 45: 555-560, 1976.

RAND R., RAND C.: *Intraspinal tumours of childhood.* Thomas, Springfield, USA pp. 1-560, 1960.

RASKAS D.S., GRAZIANO G.P., HERZENBERG J.E. ET AL.: *Osteoid osteoma and osteoblastoma of the spine.* J. Spinal Disord. 5: 204-211, 1992.

RAUHUT F., REINHARDT V., BUDACH V. ET AL.: *Intramedullary pilocytic astrocytomas. A clinical and morphological study after combined surgical and photon or neutron therapy.* Neurosurg. Rev. 12: 309-313, 1989.

RAWLINGS C., GIANGASPERO F., BURGER P.C., BULLARD D.: *Ependymomas: a clinicopathologic study.* Surg. Neurol. 29: 271-281, 1988.

REBNER M., GERBARSKI S.: *Magnetic resonance imaging of spinal cord haemangioblastoma.* AJNR 6: 287-289, 1985.

REIMER R., ONOFRIO B.: *Astrocytomas of the spinal cord in children and adolescents.* J. Neurosurg. 63: 669-675, 1985.

RENGACHARY S.S.: *Posterior and posterolateral surgical approach to the spine.* In: SUNDARESAN N. (ed.), *Tumors of the spine,* sect. C, cap. 48, pp. 488-493, 1990.

RENGACHARY S.S.: *Anterior stabilization of the cervical spine using a locking plate system.* In: RENGACHARY S.S., WILKINS R.H. (eds), *Neurosurgical Operative Atlas,* vol. 3, pp. 423-433, Williams & Wilkins, Baltimore, 1993.

RESCHE F., MOISEN J.P., MANTOURA J. ET AL.: *Haemangioblastomas, Haemangioblastomatosis and von Hippel Lindau Disease.* Advances and Technical Standard in Neurosurgery, vol. 20: 199-304, 1993; Springer-Verlag, Wien-New York.

REWCASTLE N., BERRY K: *Neoplasms of the lower spinal canal.* Neurology 14: 608-615, 1964.

RICHARDSON F.: *A report of 16 tumours of the spinal cord in children, the importance of spinal rigidity as an early sign of disease.* J. Pediatr. 57: 42-54, 1960.

RIFKINSON MANN S., WISOFF J.H., EPSTEIN F.: *The association of hydrocephalus with intramedullary spinal cord tumours: a series of 25 patients.* Neurosurgery 27: 749-754, 1990.

RISIO M., BAGLIANI C., LELI R. ET AL.: *Sacrococcigeal and vertebral chordomas. Report of three cases and review of the literature.* J. Neurosurg. Sci. 29: 211-227, 1985.

RODICHOK L., HARPER G., RUCKDESCHEL J. ET AL.: *Early diagnosis of spinal epidural metastases.* Am. J. Med. 70: 1181-1188, 1981.

ROESSNER A., MERTZE K., HEYMER B.: *Aggressive osteoblastoma.* Pathol. Res. Pract. 179: 433-436, 1985.

ROGERS M., PAILLAS J.E., DUOLAY: *Hémorragie méningée spino-cerebrale revelatrice d'une tumeur de la queue de chavez chez deux jeunes sujects.* Bull. Soc. Med. Hop. Paris 65: 37-40, 1949.

ROGERS H., LONG D., CHOU S., FRENCH L.: *Lipomas of the spinal cord and cauda equina.* J. Neurosurg. 34: 349-354, 1971.

ROMPE J., EYSEL P., HOPF C., HEINE J.: *Metastatic spinal cord compression options for surgical treatment.* Acta Neurochir. 123: 135-140, 1993.

ROSENBAUM L., NICHOLAS J.: *Early diagnosis of cervical spinal cord meningioma.* JAMA 249: 1475-1476, 1983.

ROSS D., EDWARDS M., WILSON C.: *Intramedullary neurilemomas of the spinal cord: report of two cases and review of the literature.* Neurosurgery 19: 458-464, 1986.

ROSS J., MASARYK T., MODIC M.T.: *Vertebral haemangioma: MR imaging.* Radiology 165: 165-169, 1987.

ROSSITCH E. JR, ZEIDMAN S., BURGER P. ET AL.: *Clinical and pathological analysis of spinal cord astrocytomas in children.* Neurosurgery 27: 193-196, 1990.

ROTHSTEIN T.L.: *Paraplegia resulting from rupture of previously asymptomatic intramedullary haemangioblastoma during coitus.* Ann. Neurol. 17: 5-19, 1985.

ROUX F., REY A., LECOZ P. ET AL.: *Intramedullary astrocytomas and ependymomas in adults. Are long term results altered by therapeutic tactics? Results in 23 operated cases and literature review.* Neurochirurgie 30: 99-105, 1984.

ROY-CAMILLE R., MAZEL C.H., SAILLANT G., LAPRESLE P.: *Treatment of malignant tumours of the spine with posterior instrumentation.* In: SUNDARESAN N., SCHMIDEK H.H., SCHILLER A.L., ROSENTHAL D.J.: *Tumors of the spine,* sect. C, cap. 47, pp. 473-487, 1990.

RUBIN J., DOHRMANN G.J., CHANDLER W.F.: *Intraoperative spinal ultrasonography.* Clinic Neurosurgery 34: 282-312, 1986.

RUBIN G., GORNISH M., SANDBANK J. ET AL.: *Spinal extradural angiolipoma: case report and review of the literature.* Spine 17: 719-724, 1992.

RUINI M., FILIPPI P., MAZZA S. ET AL.: *Report of four cases of osteoid osteoma and one case of benign osteoblastoma of the spine.* Riv. Neurobiol. 38: 69-72, 1992.

RUPP N.: *Zur Differenzierung von Tumoren des Spinalkanal.* Fortschr. Roentgenstr. 112: 174-182, 1970.

RUSSELL D.S.: *Capillary haemangioma of the spinal cord associated with syringomyelia.* J. Pathol. 35: 103-112, 1932.

RUSSELL D.S., RUBINSTEIN L.: *Pathology of tumours of the nervous system.* London, Edward Arnold, 3rd ed., pp. 16-19, 1971.

SACHS E. JR, HORRAX G.: *A cervical and lumbar pilonidal sinus communicating with intraspinal dermoids. Report of 2 cases and review of the literature.* J. Neurosurg. 6: 97-112, 1949.

SAKAI F., SONE S., KIYONO K.: *Intrathoracic neurogenic tumours: MR pathologic correlation.* AJR 159: 279-283, 1992.

SALVATI M., CIAPPETTA P., ARTICO M., RACO A., FORTUNA A.: *Intraspinal haemangiopericytoma: case report and review of the literature.* Neurosurg. Rev. 14: 309-313, 1991.

SANDLER H., PAPADOPOULOS S., THORNTON A. JR ET AL.: *Spinal cord astrocytomas: results of therapy.* Neurosurgery 30: 490-493, 1992.

SARPEL S., SARPEL G., YU E. ET AL.: *Early diagnosis of spinal epidural metastasis by magnetic resonance imaging.* Cancer 59: 1112-1116, 1987.

SAUNDERS R.L.: *Intramedullary epidermoid cyst associated with a dermal sinus. Case report.* J. Neurosurg. 31: 83-86, 1969.

SAVINI R., GHERLINZONI F., MORANDI M. ET AL.: *Surgical treatment of giant cell tumour of the spine. The experience at the Istituto Ortopedico Rizzoli.* J. Bone Jt. Surg. 65: 1283-1289, 1983.

SCAGLIETTI O., PANSINI A., CECCHINI M., SIMONETTI E.: *I tumori primitivi intrarachidei.* Bologna, Aulo Gaggi Editore, p. 482, 1971.

SCHIFFER J., GILBOA Y., ARLAZOROFF A.: *Epidural angiolipoma producing compression of the cauda equina.* Neurochirurgia 23: 117-120, 1980.

SCHWEITZER J.S., BATZDORF U.: *Ependymoma of the cauda equina region: diagnosis, treatment and outcome in 15 patients.* Neurosurgery 30: 202-207, 1992.

SCOTTI G., SCIALFA G., COLOMBO N., LANDONI L.: *MR imaging of intradural extramedullary tumours of the cervical spine.* J. Comput. Assisted Tomography 9: 1037-1041, 1985.

SCOTTI G., SCIALFA G., COLOMBO N. ET AL.: *Magnetic Resonance diagnosis of intramedullary tumours of the spinal cord.* Neuroradiology 29: 130-140, 1987.

SCOVILLE W.B., PALMER A.H., SAMRA K.: *The use of acrylic plastic for vertebral replacement or fixation in metastatic disesae of the spine: a technical note.* J. Neurosurg. 26: 274-276, 1967.

SEBAG G., DUBOIS J., BENIAMINOVITZ A.: *Extraosseous spinal chordoma: radiographic appearance.* AJNR 14: 205-207, 1993.

SEBASTIAN P., FISHER M., SMITH T., DAVIDSON R.: *Intramedullary spinal cord metastasis.* Surg. Neurol. 16: 336-339, 1981.

SEIFERT V., TROST H.A., STOLKE D.: *Mikrochirurgie spinaler angioblastome.* Neurochirurgia (Stuttg.) 33: 100-105, 1990.

SHAW B., MANSFIELD F., BORGES L.: *One stage posterolateral decompression and stabilization for primary and metastatic vertebral tumours in the thoracic and lumbar spine.* J. Neurosurg. 70: 405-410, 1989.

SHENKIN H., ALPERS B.: *Clinical and pathological features of the gliomas of the spinal cord.* Arch. Neurol. Psych. 52: 87-105, 1944.

SHIKATA J., YAMAMURO T., IIDA H., KOTOURA Y.: *Benign osteoblastoma of the cervical vertebra.* Surg. Neurol. 27: 381-385 1987.

SHIMIZU K., SHIKATA J., IIDA H. ET AL.: *Posterior decompression and stabilization for multiple metastatic tumours of the spine.* Spine 17: 1400-1404, 1992.

SICARD J.A.: *Les algies "d'alarme" daus les metastases cancéreuses rachidiennes.* Rev. Neurol. 39, p. 645, 1923.

SIEGAL T., SIEGAL T.: *Surgical decompression of anterior and posterior malignant epidural tumours compressing the spinal cord: a prospective study.* Neurosurgery 17: 424-432, 1985.

SIEGAL T., SIEGAL T.: *The management of malignant epidural tumours compressing the spinal cord.* In: SCHMIDEK H.H., SWEET W.H. (eds), *Operative Neurosurgical Techniques, Indications, Methods, And Results,* vol. 2, Grune And Stratton, New York, pp. 1445-1476, 1988.

SILBERGELD J., COHEN W.A., MARAVILLA K.R. ET AL.: *Supratentorial and spinal haemangioblastomas: gadolinium enhanced MR appearance with pathologic correlation.* J. Compt. Asst. Tomogr. 13: 1048-1051, 1989.

SIM F.H., DAHILIN D.C., STAUFFER R.N., LAWS E.R. JR: *Primary bone tumours simulating lumbar disc syndrome.* Spine 2: 65-74, 1977.

SIMEONE F.A.: *Spinal cord tumours in adults.* In: YOUMANS JR, *Neurological surgery,* vol. 5, pp. 3531-3547, WB Saunders Company ed., 1990.

SINSON G., ZAGER E., CHARRETTE E. ET AL.: *Metastases and spinal cord compression.* New Engl. J. Med. 327: 1953-1955, 1992.

SISTI M., STEIN B.: *Surgery of spinal meningiomas.* In: AL MEFTY O., *Meningiomas,* pp. 615-620, Raven Press, New York, 1991.

SJUTA E., KLEKAMP J., SAMII M. ET AL.: *Surgical results for intramedullary tumours with and without associated syringomyelia.* Acta Neurochir. 123: 195-199, 1993.

SLATKIN N., POSNER J.: *Management of spinal epidural metastases.* Clin. Neurosurg. 30: 698-671, 1983.

SLOOF J.L., KERNOHAN J.W., MACCARTY C.: *Primary intramedullary tumours of the spinal cord and filum terminale.* Wb Saunders Company, Philadelphia, London, 1964.

SMALTINO F., BERNINI F.P., SANTORO S.: *Computerized tomography in the diagnosis of intramedullary metastases.* Acta Neurochir. 52: 299-303, 1980.

SMALTINO F.: *Neuroradiologia*. Idelson Liviana s.r.l., 1992.

SMOKER W., GODERSKY J., KNUTZON R. ET AL.: *The role of MR imaging in evaluating metastatic spinal disease*. Am. J. Roentgenol. 149: 1241-1248, 1987.

SOLERO C., FORNARI M., GIOMBINI S. ET AL.: *Spinal meningiomas: review of 174 operated cases*. Neurosurgery 25: 133-160, 1989.

SOLINI A., PASCHERO B.: *Surgical management of spinal cord lesions due to metastases*. J. Neurosurg. Sci. 28: 201-212, 1984.

SOLINI A., PASCHERO B., ORSINI G., GUERCIO N.: *The surgical treatment of metastatic tumours of the lumbar spine*. Ital. J. Orthop. Traumatol. 11: 427-442, 1985.

SORENSEN P.S., BORGESEN S.E., ROHDE K. ET AL.: *Metastatic epidural spinal cord compression. Results of treatment and survival*. Cancer 65: 1502-1508, 1990.

SPALLONE A., DI LORENZO N., NARDI P., NOLLETTI A.: *Spinal osteochondroma diagnosed by computed tomography. Report of two cases and review of literature*. Acta Neurochir. 58: 105-114, 1981.

SPAZIANTE R., IRACE C., GAMBARDELLA A. ET AL.: *Solitary osteochondroma of the pedicle of L4 causing root compression. Case report*. J. Neurosurg. Sci. 32: 141-145, 1988.

SPAZIANTE R.: *Osteochondroma of the spine*. Neurosurgery 28: 931-932, 1991.

STEIN B.M., LEEDS N.E., TAVERAS J.M., POOL J.L.: *Meningiomas of the foramen magnum*. J. Neurosurg. 20: 740-751, 1963.

STEIN B.M.: *Surgery of intramedullary spinal cord tumours*. Clin. Neurosurg. 26: 529-542, 1979.

STEIN B.M.: *Intramedullary spinal cord tumours*. Clin. Neurosurg. 30, chapter 37, 1982.

STEIN B.M.: *Spinal intradural tumours*. In: WILKINS R.H., RENGACHARY S.S., *Neurosurgery*, vol. 2, cap. 125, Italian Edition Medical Books ed., Palermo, 1987.

STERN J., WHELAN M., CORRELL J.: *Spinal extradural meningiomas*. Surg. Neurol. 14: 155-159, 1980.

STEVENSON G.C., STONEY R.J., PERLANS R.K., ADAMS J.E.: *A transclival approach to the ventral surface of the brain stem for removal of a clivus chordoma*. J. Neurosurg. 24: 544-551, 1966.

STIMAC G., PORTER B., OLSON D. ET AL.: *Gadolinium DTPA enhanced MR imaging of spinal neoplasms: preliminary investigation and comparison with unenhanced spin echo and stir sequences*. AJNR 9: 839-846, 1988.

STRANJALIS G., JAMJOOM A., TORRENS M.: *MRI in the diagnosis of spinal extradural angiolipoma*. Br. J. Neurosurg. 6: 481-483 1992.

STRANJALIS G., TORRENS M.: *Successful removal of intramedullary spinal cord metastasis: case report*. Br. J. Neurosurg. 7: 193-195, 1993.

SUNDARESAN N., GALICICH J., CHU F., HUVOS A.: *Spinal chordomas*. J. Neurosurg. 50: 312-319, 1979.

SUNDARESAN N., GALICICH J.: *Treatment of spinal metastases by vertebral body resection*. Cancer Invest. 2: 383-397, 1984.

SUNDARESAN N., GALICICH J., BAINS M.S. ET AL.: *Vertebral body resection in the treatment of cancer involving the spine*. Cancer 53: 1393-1396, 1984.

SUNDARESAN N., GALICICH J., LANE J.: *Harrington rod stabilization for pathological fractures of the spine*. J. Neurosurg. 60: 282-286, 1984.

SUNDARESAN N., GALICICH J., LANE J. ET AL.: *Treatment of neoplastic epidural cord compression by vertebral body resection and stabilization*. J. Neurosurg. 63: 676-684, 1985.

SUNDARESAN N., ROSEN G., HUVOS A.G., KROL G.: *Combined modality treatment of osteosarcoma of the spine*. Neurosurgery 23: 714-719, 1988.

SUNDARESAN N., DIGIACINTO G.V., KROL G., HUGHES J.E.O.: *Spondylectomy for malignant tumours of the spine*. J. Clin. Oncol. 7: 1485-1491, 1989.

SUNDARESAN N., SCHILLER A.L., ROSENTHAL D.: *Osteosarcoma of the spine*. In: SUNDARESAN N., SCHMIDEK H.H., SCHILLER A.L., ROSENTHAL D.I., *Tumours of the spine diagnosis and clinical management*. Wb Saunders Company, 1990, pp. 128-145.

SUNDARESAN N., DIGIACINTO G.V., HUGHES J.E.O. ET AL.: *Treatment of neoplastic spinal cord compression: results of a prospective study*. Neurosurgery 29: 645-650, 1991.

SWANK S., BARNES R.: *Osteoid osteoma in a vertebral body. Case report*. Spine 12: 602-604, 1987.

SWEASEY T., BRUNBERG J., MCKEEVER P. ET AL.: *Cystic cervical intramedullary ependymoma with previous intracyst haemorrhage. Magnetic resonance imaging at 1,5 T.* J. Neuroimaging 4: 111-113, 1994.

SYKLAWER R., OSBORN R., KERBER C., GLASS R.: *Magnetic resonance imaging of vertebral osteoblastoma: a report of two cases.* Surg. Neurol. 34: 421-426, 1990.

SZE G., VICHANCO L.S., BRAND SAWADZKI M.N.: *Chordomas: MR imaging.* Radiology 166: 187-191, 1988.

SZE G., KROL G., ZIMMERMAN R., DECK M.: *Intramedullary disease of the spine: diagnosis using gadolinium DTPA enhanced MR imaging.* AJNR 9: 847-858, 1988.

SZE G., BRAVO S., KROL G.: *Spinal lesions: quantitative and qualitative temporal evolution of gadopentetate dimeglumine enhancement in MR imaging.* Radiology 170: 849-856, 1989.

SZE G., STIMAC G.K., BARTLETT C.: *Multicenter study of Gadopentetate dimeglumine as an MR contrast agent: evaluation in patients with spinal cord tumours.* AJNR 11: 967-974, 1990.

SZE G.: *Clinical experience with gadolinium contrast agents in spinal MR imaging.* J. Comput. Assisted Tomography 17/Suppl. 1: 8-13, 1993.

TABATABAI A., JUNGREIS C., YONAS H.: *Cervical schwannoma masquerading as a glioma: MR findings.* J. Comput. Assisted Tomography 14: 489-490, 1990.

TAKEMOTO K., MATSUMURA Y., HASHIMOTO H. ET AL.: *MR imaging of intraspinal tumours capability in histological differentiation and compartmentalization of extramedullary tumours.* Neuroradiology 30: 303-309, 1988.

TANGHETTI B., FUMAGALLI G.L., GIUNTA F. ET AL.: *Intramedullary spinal cord metastases.* J. Neurosurg. Sci. 27: 117-124, 1983.

TEKKOK I.H., ACIKGOZ B., SAGLAM S., ONOL B.: *Vertebral haemangioma symptomatic during pregnancy. Report of a case and review of the literature.* Neurosurgery 32: 302-306, 1993.

THOMAS J. , MILLER R.: *Lipomatous tumours of the spinal cord.* Mayo Clin. Proc. 48: 393-400, 1973.

THUREL R.: *Tumeurs intrarachidiennes.* J.B. Baillier et Files ed., Paris, 1964.

TILNEY F., ELSBERG C.A.: *Sensory disturbances in tumours of the cervical spinal cord: arrangement of fibres in the sensory pathways.* Arch. Neurol. Psych. 15: 444-454, 1925.

TOGNETTI F., LANZINO G., CALBUCCI F.: *Metastases of the spinal cord from remote neoplasms. Study of five cases.* Surg. Neurol. 30: 220-227, 1988.

TOKUHASHI Y., MATSUZAKI H., TORIYAMA S. ET AL.: *Scoring system for the preoperative evaluation of metastatic spine tumour prognosis.* Spine 15: 1110-1113, 1990.

TORMA T.: *Malignant tumours of the spine and the spinal extradural space. A study based on 250 histologicay verified cases.* Acta Chir. Scand., Suppl. 225: 1-176, 1957.

TOUBOUL E., ROY-CAMILLE R., GUERIN R., LEONARD P.: *Malignant epidural tumours of the spinal cord. Review of one hundred and thirty cases.* Ann. Chir. 39: 5-14, 1985.

TROST HA., SEIFERT V., STOLKE D.: *Advances in diagnosis and treatment of spinal haemangioblastomas.* Neurosurg. Rev. 16: 205-209, 1993.

URIBE BOTERO G., RUSSEL W., SUTOW W.: *Primary osteosarcoma of bone. A clinico pathologic investigation of 243 cases with necropsy studies in 54.* Am. J. Clin. Pathol. 67: 427-435, 1977.

VALK J.: *Gd DTPA in MR of spinal lesions.* AJNR 150: 1163-1168, 1988.

VAN DER SLUIS R., GURR K., JOSEPH M.: *Osteochondroma of the lumbar spine: an unusual cause of sciatica.* Spine 17: 1519-1521, 1992.

VARMA D.G.K., MOULOPOULOS A., SARA A.: *MR imaging of extracranial nerve sheath tumours.* J. Comp. Ass. Tomogr. 16: 448-453, 1992.

VENKATARAMANA N., KOLLURI V., NARAYANA SWAMY K. ET AL.: *Exophytic gliomas of the spinal cord.* Acta Neurochir. 107: 44-46, 1990.

VERBIEST H.: *Neurogenic intermittens claudicatio.* In: VINKEN P.J., BRUYN G.W. (eds), *Handbook of Clinical Neurology,* Amsterdam, North-Holland, vol. 20, pp. 661-807, 1976.

VERNET O., ALAILI R., DE TRIBOLET N.: *Les emhorrhagies sous-arachnoidiennes spinales.* Scweiz Med. Wschr. 116: 781-785, 1986.

VIALE E.: *Intramedullary epidermoid tumours.* Neurochirurgia (Stuttg.) 20: 116-118, 1977.

VISCIANI A., SAVOIARDO M., BALESTRINI M., SOLERO C.: *Iatrogenic intraspinal epidermoid tumor: Myelo CT and MRI diagnosis.* Neuroradiology 31: 273-275, 1989.

VITZTHUM E.H., KRUMBHOLZ S., WILLENBERG E.: *Problem of the early recognition of spinal cord tumours.* Zentralbl. Neurochir. 43: 151-215, 1982.

VLES J., GRUBBEN C., VAN OOY A., WEIL E.: *Holocord astrocytomas in childhood.* Clin. Neurol. Neurosurg. 92: 361-364, 1990.

VON HANWEHR R., APUZZO M., AHMADI J., CHANDRASOMA P.: *Thoracic spinal angiomyolipoma: case report and literature review.* Neurosurgery 16: 406-411, 1985.

WATABE T., AZUMA T.: *T1 and T2 measurements of meningiomas and neurinomas before and after Gd DTPA.* AJNR 10: 463-470, 1989.

WATANABE M., KIHARA Y., MATSUDA Y., SHIBATA T.: *Benign osteoblastoma in the vertebral body of the thoracic spine: a case report.* Spine 17: 1432-1433, 1992.

WEBB J., CRAIG M., KERNOHAN J.: *Intraspinal neoplasm in the cervical region.* J. Neurosurg. 10: 360-366, 1953.

WENG QUING H., SHI JU Z., YU XIA L. ET AL.: *Statistical analysis of central nervous system tumours in China.* J. Neurosurg. 56: 555-564, 1982.

WERTHEIMER P., ALLÈGRE G., GARDE A.: *Les tumeurs épendymaires de la moelle et du filum terminale.* Rev. Neurol. 82: 153-162, 1950.

WHITE W., FRASER R.: *Cervical spinal cord lipoma with extension into the posterior fossa.* Neurosurgery 12: 460-462, 1983.

WHITMER G., DAVIS R., BELL D.: *Hanging head sign as a presenting feature of spinal cord neoplasms: a report of four cases.* J. Pediatr. Orthop. 13: 322-324, 1993.

WILLIAMS A., HAUGHTON V., POJUNAS K. ET AL.: *Differentiation of intramedullary neoplasms and cysts by MR.* AJR 149: 159-163, 1987.

WIPPOLD F., CITRIN C., BARKOVICH A., SHERMAN J.: *Evaluation of MR in spinal dysraphism with lipoma: comparison with metrizamide computed tomography.* Pediatr. Radiol. 17: 184-188, 1987.

WISOFF H., SUZUKI Y., LLEENA J., FINE D.: *Extramedullary haemangioblastoma of the spinal cord. Case report.* J. Neurosurg. 48: 461-464, 1978.

WISS D.: *An unusual cause of sciatica and back pain: ependymoma of the cauda equina. Case report.* J. Bone Joint Surg. 64: 772-773, 1982.

WOLTMAN H.W., KEROHAN J.W., ADSON A.W., CRAIG W.: *Intramedullary tumours of spinal cord and gliomas of intradural portion of filum terminale. Fate of patients who have these tumours.* Arch. Neurol. Psych. 65, p. 378, 1951.

WONG D., FORNASIER V., MACNAB I.: *Spinal metastases: the obvious, the occult, and the impostors.* Spine 15: 1-4, 1990.

WYBURN-MASON R.: *The vascular abnormalities and tumours of the spinal cord and its membranes.* London, H. Kimpton, 1943.

YABLON J.: *Osteochondroma of the vertebral column.* Neurosurgery 27: 659-660, 1990.

YAMASHITA K., FUJI T., NAKAI T. ET AL.: *Extradural spinal angiolipoma: report of a case studied with MRI.* Surg. Neurol. 39: 49-52 1993.

YAMAZAKI M., IKOTA T., OHKATA N. ET AL.: *A case of spinal cord glioblastoma multiforme.* Neurol. Surg. 20: 85-89, 1992.

YASARGIL M.G., ANTIC J., LACIGA R. ET AL.: *The microsurgical removal of intramedullary spinal haemangioblastomas: report of twelve cases and a review of the literature.* Surg. Neurol. 6: 141-148, 1976.

YOKUM T., LILE R., SCHULTZ G.: *Acquired spinal stenosis secondary to an expanding thoracic vertebral haemangioma.* Spine 18: 299-305, 1993.

YOSHIZAWA M., O'BRIEN J.P., SMITH W. ET AL.: *The neuropathology of intervertebral disc removed for low back pain.* J. Pathol. 132: 95-104, 1980.

YOUNG R., POST E., KING G.: *Treatment of spinal epidural metastases. Randomized prospective comparison of laminectomy and radiotherapy.* J. Neurosurg. 53: 741-748, 1980.

YU Y., CROCKARD H., SMITH J., HARRIES B.: *Extraspinal ependymoma at the cervicothoracic junction.* Surg. Neurol. 17: 160-162, 1982.

YUH W., FLICKINGER F., BARLOON T., MONTGOMERY W.: *MR imaging of unusual chordomas.* J. Comput. Asst. Tomogr. 12: 30-35, 1988.

ZULCH K.: *Pathology and natural history of mass lesion in the spinal cord, its covers and in the neighbouring vertebral column.* Radiolog., 20: 459-465, 1980.

Finito di stampare nel mese di aprile 1997
dalla Everprint, Carugate (MI)